SAVING FACE

SAVING FACE

My Victory Over Skin Cancer

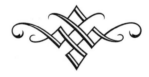

CAROLYN SHUCK

Introduction by Hubert T. Greenway, M.D.

Paul S. Eriksson, *Publisher*
Forest Dale, Vermont

5 4 3   2   1

Library of Congress Cataloging-in-Publication Data

Shuck, Carolyn.
    Saving face : my victory over skin cancer / Carolyn Shuck ; foreword by Hubert
T. Greenway.
        p.   cm.
    Includes index.
    ISBN 0-8397-7340-4 (hardcover)
        1. Shuck, Carolyn--Health. 2. Basal cell carcinoma--Patients--California--
Biography. I. Title.
    RC280.S5 S55 2000
    362.1'9699477'0092--dc21
    [B]   00-037555

Design by Eugenie S. Delaney

*To the two physicians primarily responsible for saving
my face and my life—Dr. Fredrick E. Mohs, who successfully
removed my facial skin cancer, and Dr. Edmund Klein,
who immunized my body so that it has fought off
any more skin cancer since 1974.*

CONTENTS

ACKNOWLEDGMENTS

Writing this book has been a hard and rigorous but pleasant experience—one I have greatly enjoyed. I have worked on it for many years for two main reasons: 1.) As a therapeutic message for myself, I felt it important to record my struggle against skin cancer, and 2.) I wanted to pass on to others suffering from this same condition the knowledge I have gained.

I am extremely grateful to Dr. Hubert Greenway for his medical care and friendship over the years, and for writing the Introduction; and to my son Ted and his wife Marsha, for their invaluable assistance in proofreading, typing, and helping in the details of getting the book published.

My warm thanks to Jack Pickering, whose editing skills, advice and comments I have sought and found most helpful. I also want to thank my publishers—especially Paul Eriksson himself who has helped tremendously.

I hope I've given credit where credit is due, and haven't neglected those to whom I owe so much.

INTRODUCTION

When Carolyn Shuck asked me to write the Introduction for her book, I was delighted. Each of us has our own story to tell, and her journey in dealing with the devastating skin cancer in the middle of her face is one of courage, persistence, and strength.

We met years ago, following my skin-cancer-fellowship training with Fred Mohs, M.D., at the University of Wisconsin in Madison. During my time with him I assisted in treating 200 patients a month for skin cancers including basal cell carcinoma, squamous cell carcinoma, malignant melanoma, and others. Many of these patients were wonderful individuals who came from all over the world to seek care from Dr. Mohs who used the technique he had developed to trace the cancer and achieve the maximum cure rate.

Carolyn had had a similar experience years before my days in Madison, when she sought out the wonderful Dr. Mohs to care for her cancer. After my training with him, I returned to La Jolla, California (which is about as far as one can get from Madison), and met Carolyn who said it was no longer necessary for her to travel to Madison for follow-up visits. She would be under my care. Truly, Fred Mohs is one of medicine's greats, having researched and developed innovations in his technique, treating thousands of patients while doing so, and finally sharing his knowledge freely by training physicians like me who now train others. Thus I became Carolyn Shuck's physician.

She and her husband DeWitt (along with others) enticed me to join Scripps Clinic and Research Foundation so patients could be treated in La Jolla. She continued her follow-ups and, as expected, has had no evidence of cancer in the area treated by Dr. Mohs.

Cancer is a devastating diagnosis to give to the patient. Questions immediately arise, such as "Are you sure?"; "Am I going to die?"; "Could there be a mistake in the diagnosis?" and many others. While basal cell carcinoma skin cancer normally does not metastasize (perhaps we see in our clinic one or two cases a year that do), it can be extremely aggressive and devastating, especially if not completely cured at first. Such was the case with Carolyn many years ago. She could not have imagined the extent of spread of skin cancer in the middle of her face. The middle of our face is our "passport." This is *you* and how the world sees you. Just look in the mirror and imagine yourself without most of your nose. How would you feel and cope?

The story of Carolyn's experience with Dr. Mohs involves not only her treatment. Also vital to it are her attempts and ability to cope. She became part of the "family" (Dr. Mohs and his staff, headed by his nurse, Rachel), as she now had to deal with the loss of the middle of her face in order to eliminate the cancer before it tracked back into the skull and brain. Her worst nightmares seemed to be coming true. Subsequently the long ordeal of rebuilding had to take place and this, too, was complex and challenging for all involved. Finally the question of follow-up and "Are we sure we got it all?" had to be dealt with so life could go on.

Today Carolyn continues to be an inspiration to my life and to the lives of others. After a case similar to hers in which I had to remove a large portion of the nose of a wonderful young woman named Liz, I asked Carolyn if she would help—get involved—as Liz would have to deal with many issues she herself had faced. Her involvement was and still is inspiring. The two women see each other frequently, and Carolyn absolutely had "been there, done that" and survived, for Liz to see as she confronted her own facial cancer.

I am amazed at how we learn and are influenced by those with whom we come in contact. Many years ago I was among a number of guests of Carolyn and DeWitt Shuck as they entertained Dr. Mohs. I realized then that, really, we are all "family."

Carolyn Shuck's story is very special. I encourage you to enjoy, to cry, to believe, and to gain from it.

Hubert T. Greenway, M.D.
Chairman, Dermatology and Cutaneous Surgery
Medical Director, Skin and Cosmetic Surgery Center
Scripps Clinic

SAVING FACE

PROLOGUE

On the 23rd of September, 1970, summer came to a sudden end in Madison, Wisconsin. The temperature dropped from the eighties to the forties in a matter of hours. Just the day before, at home in Minneapolis, I'd gone grocery shopping in my yellow golf dress and barefoot sandals. Now, as I struggled in the gusty fall wind to open the heavy front door to the Ivy Inn in Madison, I was glad I'd brought along my tweed coat.

Once inside, I went right to the bar.

"A martini to go."

A woman at the bar looked at the thick white bandage that covered my nose.

"Do you think it's wise to drink so soon following anesthesia?"

"I haven't had any anesthesia. That's why I need the martini."

At the front desk I picked up the key to Room 121. Carrying the martini—very carefully—I walked down a long narrow hallway to my room. Once inside I locked the door and leaned against it. A day from hell, all eight hours of it. I'd had to keep my suffering to myself.

Finally, alone.

The martini went on the bedside table. The novel I'd tried to read all day slammed onto the dresser. I kicked off my shoes. One hit the wall. Flung my coat and best bag onto the floor in a heap, downed the martini, and crashed onto the bed. There I stayed for two long hours.

I didn't dare cry—my nose would run, I'd have to blow it, and that would hurt. The walls of my room seemed very thin. I could only moan. But I thrashed around on the bed, kicking and pounding at the pillows and mattress. How I wanted to *scream.*

Only two months ago Dr. Frederick E. Mohs had removed deep, spreading cancers from my forehead and chin. Dr. Mohs was a world-renowned expert in chemosurgery. He had ended my problem. I'd be okay.

I was wrong. If this new cancer were as bad as those others were, there wouldn't be much of my nose left when he finished. My nose was small and delicate, the tip finely chiseled. I'd always considered it my best feature. What had I got myself into? Great God in Heaven, not—surely not—a deformed nose. Impossible to overlook, right there in the middle of my face, the first thing people saw when they looked at me. No clothing could ever cover it.

I punched the pillow and kicked some more.

If only this were one of those nightmares when you're lost and can't find your way home, or being chased by mad dogs, or falling off a cliff. You awaken, crying in terror, to the sweet realization that you've been dreaming.

But I couldn't wake up. And it wasn't a dream. Instead, it was the beginning of a seven-year struggle to save my face.

1.

INITIATION

I t was the month of June, 1970. Had anyone asked me how I was on any of those long, golden days in my fiftieth year, I'd have told them I believed myself to be one of the most fortunate people ever to inhabit the face of the earth.

For twenty years I'd been married to DeWitt Shuck, as outstanding a husband as he was a businessman. Our large, beautiful house in Minneapolis overlooked a lake, the scene changing from a Manet watercolor in the summer to a Currier and Ives print in the winter. John and Ted, our handsome college-age sons, both had brilliant minds and solid values—demonstrably, even allowing for maternal bias. Our ten-year-old daughter Ellen was the sugar loaf angel on our cake.

Of course there were the daily irritations, but rarely did more than a fluffy white cloud float across my bright blue sky.

For years I'd done volunteer work with poverty-level women, listened to them, talked with them, spent time in their homes. The stark contrast between their lives and mine made me think about just how lucky I *was*.

Basal cell skin cancer had plagued me since I was thirty-two, but I saw it as more a nuisance than any cause for real concern. I'd see my dermatologist every three months, have little things cut out and promptly forget about them. Before going out on the golf course I applied the best available sunscreen for that time. It wasn't very effective, but I hoped it would cut down on the length of my dermatology visits.

Doctors had, over the years, encouraged this nonchalant attitude. "You'll probably have forty more of these during your lifetime," said the dermatologist who'd removed my very first tiny basal cell skin cancer from my forehead eighteen years before. The basis for his prediction was the X-ray treatments I'd received as an adolescent. X-rays were a popular acne cure in the 1920's and 1930's. Dermatologists did not learn until years later that nine out of ten patients receiving X-ray treatments for acne developed skin cancer.

But my dermatologist seemed perfectly confident that medical science could cure the disease it had caused. And so, without a qualm, I spent weeks on the beach in Acapulco every winter and went deep sea fishing with DeWitt off the coast of Baja. And each time we came back from Mexico, my dermatologist would remove a few more small basal cell skin cancers.

By June of 1970, I'd been out on the golf course for a month. A few marshy places served to remind us that the course had only recently emerged from its deep, white blanket. It felt great to be out running around in my golf dress and sandals, not all bundled up in coats and boots.

During my annual checkup at a well-regarded clinic in May, I'd complained about a crusting place on my nose that tended to bleed at times. A staff physician there had cauterized it, but it still troubled me a little. And so, when I read about research on a new sunscreen now being conducted at the University of Minnesota, I was immediately interested.

"Take a look at this." I passed the newspaper page to DeWitt. "Maybe this Dr. Lynch could get me some of this stuff—might be great for golf days this summer."

DeWitt shrugged. "Whatever you think. But if you go today, be back before the traffic gets bad. Remember, we're going to the Peytons' for dinner this evening."

"No problem. This shouldn't take long at all."

I washed off all my makeup and drove to St. Paul to see Dr. Francis Lynch, a prominent dermatologist on the staff of the University of Minnesota.

"Can't you get me on the guinea pig list for the new sunscreen?" I asked him.

He ignored my question. Instead, he looked very carefully at a cancer scar on my forehead and one on my chin.

"You know," he said, "these old places don't look healthy. I'd like you to see Dr. Fred Mohs—he's in Madison, Wisconsin."

"Can't you just take care of them yourself?"

"No, I want you to see Mohs. He's a specialist in the field. I'd like to have him take a look at them."

I smiled. "If I'm going to get to go somewhere, why don't you send me to New York or San Francisco? I don't know a soul in Wisconsin." Dr. Lynch overlooked my feeble joke.

"Dr. Mohs has developed a specific technique for removing skin cancers. The procedure is accepted now and he's even trained some others in his method, but he himself is still the seat of all wisdom."

"Why don't you just send me to a plastic surgeon?"

"A plastic surgeon would remove far more tissue, taking some healthy skin around the cancer to get a margin of safety." He fingered the scars. "Dr. Mohs' procedure will get out all of a skin cancer, but not cut out any healthy tissue. The way these old scars look now, I'd say the original removals weren't complete. Cancer is probably still active in those areas."

"How long do you think I'll have to stay there?"

"Only two or three days."

"Is it the kind of thing . . . do you think my husband needs to go with me?"

"I don't think so," he said, and had his secretary call for an appointment.

DeWitt and I talked over everything Dr. Lynch had said and agreed that he wouldn't be sending me to Wisconsin without good reason. I telephoned Dr. Mohs' secretary in Madison and asked her to book a room for me at the Ivy Inn.

"I've heard it's very nice," I said.

"It is. Also very expensive. You could stay at Mandel House— it's only a block from our offices, and an air-conditioned room is seven dollars a night."

"Sounds like a bargain. Make my reservation there for Monday, July 27. And what time is my appointment?"

"Dr. Mohs doesn't take appointments. Get here as soon as you can. It's first come, first served. You can take the shuttle bus from the airport to University Hospitals."

"What's his office number?"

"If you ask at the reception desk just inside the lobby, they'll tell you where to come."

"Could I ask what your name is?"

"Mary Jane."

"Thanks a lot, Mary Jane. I'll see you next week."

On July 27 I flew to Madison, fortified with scotch and in

reasonably high spirits anyway. This would be a vacation of sorts—I could go to a movie, maybe even an R-rated movie. Something not suitable for ten-year-olds.

It first struck me this trip might not prove altogether festive when I looked at the entry door to Dr. Mohs' offices and read the large block letters on its opaque window: CHEMOSURGERY. I'd never seen the word spelled out before—had never once thought of my basal cell cancer removals as *surgeries*.

I entered the open doorway, and even at this early morning hour it was warm and muggy inside. The building wasn't air-conditioned; only a small electric fan moved the air. I went to a small office off the waiting room.

"Mary Jane?"

"Yes?"

"I'm Mrs. Shuck. I called you last week from Minneapolis. You told me to just come in at 7:30 a.m. today, as it was first-come-first-served. Am I first?"

"I don't think so." She smiled. "I'll introduce you to Rachel, Dr. Mohs' nurse."

Rachel smiled, shook my hand and nodded toward the waiting room.

"Just find a chair; we'll call you in shortly."

The waiting room seemed ridiculously small for one in a large state-supported hospital. It was already filled to capacity, and at least twenty more patients were spilling over into the outer hospital hallway. The hall was lined with straight, stainless steel chairs—hopefully enough to accommodate the overflow.

I looked around me. The patients who had pink Band-Aid-type plasters on their faces, necks, or arms, looked like patients I'd seen in other dermatologists' offices. I'd often looked the same way myself. But there were others, with larger white bandages covering more of their exposed skin. Unlike the small-bandage patients, these were not reading or chatting. Their faces looked solemn, and I wondered if their wounds were painful.

I listened to conversations and asked a few questions. Many of these patients, I learned, had come to see Dr. Mohs from distant parts of the country. It seemed that Dr. Lynch had been right—although I wasn't in a plush office in New York or San Francisco, I was, as he'd said, at the seat of all wisdom.

When Rachel finally called me to an inner office, I sat down in what looked like a barber's chair. Dr. Mohs, a large silent man, was wearing what appeared to be a butcher's apron and had some sort of miner's lamp on his head. He struck me as relaxed and amiable, though he just nodded and smiled when Rachel introduced me. Perhaps it was the deep-furrowed laugh lines around his eyes that made him immediately seem a kind and comfortable man, just the sort you could imagine as a costumed Santa. Not a skinny little Santa, but a good, hearty one.

He looked over my face, then daubed something on several places. It stung a bit but not enough to matter.

"What are you doing? I asked.

"Getting these places ready for biopsy."

"Could I see the stuff you're daubing on?"

"Sure." It was a black paste, about the consistency of peanut butter.

"What's it called?"

"Zinc chloride."

"It isn't going to hurt, is it?"

Rachel gave me a quick glance and started sticking on pink bandages.

"You want us to treat you, but you don't want us to hurt you," she said.

Of course I didn't want to be hurt. I wasn't crazy. Was she trying to tell me something?

"Come back at two o'clock," she said, and she handed me a prescription for pain pills.

"Oh, I probably won't need these." I nonchalantly waved the small white paper, not wanting her to think I was a wimp.

"Maybe you should get the prescription filled. Just in case."

The waiting room was so full, I didn't feel like taking up their time with more questions. I wanted to know what, exactly, Dr. Mohs was up to—and couldn't remember his saying much of anything. Well, he had said "biopsy." I thanked them both and left.

I had four hours to kill with pink Band-Aids on my face. Not that I was in the least embarrassed. Over the past twenty years I'd had enough small cancers removed that the Band-Aid look had become almost normal. When we'd lived in Iowa, a good friend had once called across the room at a party, "There she is, plastered again."

I found the hospital dispensary, handed over the prescription, and got back a bottle of inch-long yellow capsules. I put them in my purse, wondering how I'd ever swallow them.

"What are these things, anyway?" I asked the pharmacist.

"Codempiral. A combination of codeine and emperin."

"Oh. Well, thanks." And I was off to Mandel House.

There was no lobby, just a little provisions counter on the main floor. The young man behind the counter handed me the key to Room 227.

"Here you go," he said. "And you'll need some sheets, towels, and a wash cloth."

I trundled upstairs with my gear and let myself into my room. Where was the TV? Where was the toilet paper? Maybe I had to supply my own. After all, they were selling it in that grocery store downstairs. But the thing that seemed strangest was the pay tele-phone on the wall.

I've always considered a little dust to be one of life's better-ignored problems, but this place was so grimy my hands were char-coal-gray after simply unpacking and plugging in my little electric typewriter. (I'd brought it along to catch up on back correspon-dence between movies.) I used my hand towel to wipe off the dresser and table tops. Now the hand towel was charcoal gray, so I couldn't use it to wipe out the tub.

At noon, I went downstairs where the grocery clerk leaned against the counter.

"Is there a good place to eat lunch around here?"

"Sure, there's a drug store a block away that serves great food." He pointed in the direction of Dr. Mohs' offices. "It's right on your way to the Hospital."

I ate a grilled cheese sandwich and some limp coleslaw in a fluted paper cup, then headed back to Dr. Mohs'.

Two boulevards, heavy with traffic, separated me from his office. I punched a button and when the green "WALK" sign came on, started across the boulevard—only to see the sign start blinking "DON'T WALK" when I was halfway across. What was I supposed to do, stand stock-still with cars three abreast gunning for me? I ran across, wishing I'd worn tennis shoes.

At two o'clock I was seated in Dr. Mohs' outer hallway, now more crowded than ever. While I was there, two patients on gurneys were wheeled down from the hospital upstairs. One man had a large bandage covering half his face and neck. He looked so alone, I almost rushed up to squeeze his hand, which lay on top of the sheet.

I didn't do it, of course. I couldn't. The thought of what that bandage might be covering made me swallow hard.

"Come in, Mrs. Shuck," Rachel said. Once I was back in the barber chair, Dr. Mohs pared away the chemically impregnated sections to examine under his microscope. It didn't hurt at all. Why had he bothered to prescribe those yellow horse-capsules?

Rachel gently stuck on a few bandages.

"Wait outside for the results. They'll be ready in about an hour."

I read a newspaper someone had left in a chair, but I was bored without a good book. I decided to cast the scene I'd just lived through. Walter Matthau would play Dr. Mohs, Debbie Reynolds would play Rachel, and Carol Channing would play me.

"How many of those places you tested were cancerous?" I asked when Rachel called me back in.

"Only two. Your forehead and chin."

The doctor reapplied chemical to those areas. It still didn't hurt.

"Come back tomorrow morning," Rachel said.

"What time?"

"Any time after seven."

I decided to go right back to Mandel House. The room might leave much to be desired, but I wanted to get back to my typewriter. The last letter I'd written was a Christmas thank-you, and it was practically July.

Before I reached the lobby, a burning pain ripped through my forehead and chin. I rushed for the drinking fountain, rummaged through my handbag, found the bottle, and gulped down one heavenly yellow capsule.

I staggered back through "WALK" and "DON'T WALK" signals to Mandel House, fell against the elevator button, and let myself into Room 227. I lay down, wished I had a pillow. Didn't care.

Burned . . . Burned . . . Burned . . .

I woke myself up snoring. Snoring? Only DeWitt snores.

I looked at my watch. Almost six in the evening. I gently touched my chin and forehead. The burning had stopped, thank heaven.

Going down in the elevator, I met two women. One, who had a large bandage covering her nose, attempted a smile when she saw the pink plasters on my forehead and chin.

"I see we go to the same doctor," I said.

"Yours are so little," the woman said. "Dr. Mohs has had to remove a lot of my nose."

"Oh. How awful."

"I'm Margaret Murphy. I've been here two weeks. It's been horrible—without my sister here, I'd never have made it."

"Now Dr. Mohs says she'll have to have it rebuilt by a plastic surgeon," her sister said. "He recommended one here."

"We're from South Dakota," Margaret said, "and I don't want to stay in Madison any longer. I want to go home."

"I don't blame you. After two weeks here, I'd be dying to go home too. Maybe there'll be a good plastic surgeon out your way."

My heart ached for her. What could be worse than losing your nose?

"Would you like to have dinner together?" I said.

"Sure," the sister said. "I've heard there's a steak house on the outskirts of Madison that's air conditioned." The heat had been stifling all day and the evening didn't promise much of an improvement.

We hailed a taxi. Before the ride was over I could see that Margaret was not only distraught, she needed and demanded perpetual consolation. She couldn't let the conversation shift even momentarily to another topic.

When her sister said, "It's almost as easy to go back home on the train as it is to fly," Margaret said, "I think I'll try taking two codempirals tonight to see if I'll sleep any better."

I really felt sorry for her sister. Her role in this awful drama was going to be hard, in some ways harder than Margaret's. I was lucky. Rachel said my removals would just heal in and any leftover scars would be minor.

2.

EXCAVATION

I understood Dr. Mohs' technique much better after my first day's experience on Monday. Rachel having explained the procedure as a series of logical steps really helped.

First he applied a chemical to any skin areas that appeared cancerous. After an hour or two the chemical deadened the skin.

He pared off enough tissue from the chemically stained areas to examine under his microscope. Then, wherever examination showed still active cancer, he applied more of the chemical. But he applied the chemical *only* to that area of the skin slice that showed cancer.

He would keep paring off and examining very thin slices of skin until the bottom of a skin slice proved cancer-free.

I felt much more confident the next morning. I knew what to expect, and even a little knowledge is strong protection against fear and uncertainty.

My new-found understanding extended to the pain I had felt—and would feel again. The paring off of tissue didn't hurt at all because the chemical had deadened the skin. The application of the chemical, even to raw places where skin had been sliced off before, didn't hurt at first. No, the real pain wouldn't start until I was approximately ninety feet away from his office.

Then the burning would begin, and last about two hours. What made it even worse was that you couldn't go douse your face in a sink full of cold water. Enter the yellow capsule, which would render the pain dull and far away.

The problem was, the yellow capsules made me want desperately to sit down anywhere I was: in the hallway, in the middle of Dr. Mohs' operating parlor, in the hospital lobby, in the middle of a busy street, "WALK—DON'T WALK" signs be damned.

I turned to aspirin. During a painful period, I'd go to the hospital lobby and gulp down three of them at the drinking fountain. If I were due back in his office in a few hours, I'd curl up in an overstuffed lobby chair. If I didn't have to come back until morning, at least I could safely cross the busy boulevard that separated his office from Mandel House without feeling the crosswalk was suddenly a good place for a nap.

The pain lasted almost precisely two hours—I'd keep a constant check on my watch. It was a relief to know that after the hour hand had circled twice, the pain would be gone. When an end to suffering can be predicted, it is far more bearable. Again, a little knowledge can be a powerful shield.

As each cutting went deeper, the application of the chemical became more and more painful. Just before one cutting, I mentioned it to Dr. Mohs.

"You know, you're a very sneaky man."

"Why's that?"

"You've got this whole thing timed so it doesn't hurt till I'm exactly ninety feet away from your assigned space in this hospital and your shins are safe."

"Pretty clever."

He did cuttings on my forehead and chin Monday, Tuesday, and Wednesday. By Thursday noon he was finished. When I looked in the mirror above his office sink I was appalled. I had a hole in my forehead about two inches in diameter—some Las Vegas gambler could have dropped three silver dollars into it. The hole in my chin was about half that size.

"These places will fill in after about six weeks," he said. "There'll be only minor scarring."

It was hard to believe. But perhaps because he was a man of so few words, when he did say something, I believed him. I left his office reassured.

My eyes were swollen, and large fluid-filled bags hung under them. I'd lugged that silly typewriter all that way for nothing. I couldn't have typed or seen an X-or-R movie if someone had led me into the theater and plopped me down in the front row.

I called DeWitt's office and his secretary answered. "Either Mr. Shuck or I will meet you at the airport gate in Minneapolis."

I thought I could get that far.

I took another look at myself in the mirror.

Do I want DeWitt to think I'm pitiful? Or should I crawl to the drug store and get dark glasses? I thought of Margaret's sister.

I got the glasses.

On my return flight to Minneapolis, I thought about how different my experience over the last few days had been from what I'd anticipated. The trip was to have been a small holiday with a few bothersome trips to a famous doctor for skin cancer treatment squeezed in. But I'd envisioned his office to be like that of other noted specialists with maybe a dozen patients seated comfortably in an attractively furnished waiting room. I'd been certain I'd be given a local anesthetic. "Nowadays even dentistry is painless," I'd say to myself.

I sat by a woman who was going to Kansas City to see her new grandchild. She nodded toward the large white bandages that covered my forehead and chin. "Have you been in a car wreck?"

"No. I ran into a doctor's scalpel." I turned to face her. I had to tell someone. "I've just had one of the most bizarre experiences of my life. I stayed in a hotel with a grocery store for a lobby and bought my own soap and toilet paper. When I checked out, at least it wasn't in the grocery store, but it was in Room 302 where I gave $23 for a three-night stay to a young woman rolling out pizza dough on top of an old sewing machine cabinet. One thing is sure: the price was right."

She asked, "What kind of surgery did you have?"

"Skin cancer."

"Oh, my sister has those. She just ignores them."

Heavens. Had I been through this outlandish experience for no good reason? I'd have to ask Dr. Mohs when I went back.

When DeWitt met me at the airport, his eyes widened, then he frowned. He didn't give me his usual hug, but squeezed my hand. At first I thought he was irritated because he'd had to look around for me and feared I'd given his secretary the wrong flight number.

But when I told him I was to go back to Madison in ten days, he shook his head. "Next time, I'm going with you. When we get home, you go straight to bed."

I couldn't help smiling a little. I knew his gruffness was a cover for the concern he felt.

The house was empty, the children were all away at camp. The boys were having fun as counselors and Ellen was suffering pangs of homesickness. I was glad for some solitude. Glad too that they were spared the sight of Dr. Mohs' handiwork.

The chemical had made my stomach queasy, and the shock of

the ordeal had left me weak. I went to bed for several days with my radio, eyes too swollen to read or watch TV.

I was supposed to apply mercurochrome to the wounds each day. But the first day I removed the large white gauze dressings and just dropped back into bed. The sight of those wounds uncovered was too much.

I was glad Kay Dawson was there. She'd been our housekeeper for four years and we'd become good friends.

"Good God," she said when she saw me, "With that hole in my head, I'd stay right there in bed until it heals."

"Think you could help me with these bandages, Kay?"

She didn't answer and I knew she wasn't deaf.

No chance of her helping me out. Damn. Well, it had to be done. Come on, Carolyn. Mohs' excavations aren't for sissies.

Very, very carefully, I went over the wounds with a mercurochrome-soaked Q-tip. To my surprise, it didn't hurt at all.

When my ten days "off duty" were over, DeWitt went with me to Madison. At Dr. Mohs' place they seated him in the outer hallway.

"I see you've brought along your bodyguard," Dr. Mohs said as I sat once more in his barber chair.

The idea of DeWitt as a burly bodyguard made me laugh. It wasn't that he was incapable of warding off danger, but he was always so distinguished. Even now, he sat among the informally dressed patients in Dr. Mohs' hallway reading his *Wall Street Journal*, flawlessly groomed and impeccably tailored. The idea also kept me from thinking about what was going to happen.

Until Dr. Mohs picked up a small pair of scissors. I sat there stiff as a board while he deftly clipped off the wound's outer crusts. But it didn't hurt, at least not much.

"Come back in a month," he said, "around September 9. I want to remove some bone behind the forehead scar."

Bone? Wants to remove some *bone*? Good grief.

"Will it be bad?"

"Not too bad."

"Can I have novocaine?"

"I'll give you a topical anesthetic."

Why did asking for an anesthetic make me feel as though I'd asked for a double bourbon at a Women's Christian Temperance Union meeting?

We went to Colorado to pick up Ellen at camp. She had her gear packed and was ready to leave. She was also in tears.

"Honey, why in the world are you crying?"

"I'll miss Becky and Angela and . . . and Kim . . . ."

"What about all those letters pleading to come home early?"

Ted, a counselor at camp that summer, came up to us. He kissed me, shook his father's hand, then put his arm around Ellen's shoulder and pulled her close.

"She's liked it a lot better lately, haven't you?"

Ellen wiped her eyes on her wrist. "Uh huh."

"Are you ready to leave and go down to the Garden of the Gods Club?" I asked. "Maybe drive up Pikes Peak?"

"Sure". She sniffed one last time, then looked closely at my face. "Say, what did Dr. Mohs *do* to you, anyway?"

"He had to remove a lot of skin cancer, but it'll heal up in about six weeks."

"Oh, Mom, I'm real sorry. Did you have to be brave?"

I laughed. "Yes, sweetie, a little bit brave."

"I'm sorry, Mom," Ted said. "I love you, you know."

"I know."

I gazed into the luminous blue eyes of my son, protective of his sister, handsome inside and out . . . .

And remembered.

I *was*, all things considered, the luckiest woman in the world.

The other thing we did on my month off was vacation in Colorado. Shanghaied into driving up Pikes Peak with DeWitt and Ellen, I jumped out of the car at the halfway house.

"What are you *doing*, Mother?"

"Ellen, get out here with me if you have half a grain of sense."

DeWitt and I had recently been forced off a highway while going seventy miles an hour. We had rolled over and over into a gully, finally coming to a halt on our roof when our fenders stuck in a mud bank. We'd been wearing our seat belts, so neither of us was injured. But I was still scared silly driving up and down small hills, and almost hysterical on high mountains.

At the halfway house, I read a pamphlet, "Tips for Driving up Pikes Peak," and realized that Dewitt hadn't followed a single one of them. I'd never seen him put the car in low—and I'd opened my eyes at least twice.

On the way back down the mountain, I kept my eyes shut and vowed not to peek. And fantasized about my upcoming trip to Madison to have forehead bone removed via knife. Soon after this death-defying vacation, I'd be back again in Dr. Mohs' operating chair.

Safe again.

On the early morning flight to Madison two weeks later, whenever I thought of the ordeal ahead of me I simply reminded myself that I *could* be driving up Pikes Peak.

Once in his office, I had all the confidence in the world. In the past, Dr. Mohs had hurt me only by delayed timing, and this was not to be "too bad."

I relaxed into the reclining barber chair—and clutched its arms.

"Topical anesthetic, remember?"

Rachel painted some on.

When Dr. Mohs entered the room I was lying nearly horizontal. He carefully placed himself behind my head so that I could not possibly see his weapon.

I swear it was a hammer and chisel. It felt as if my forehead was a window and he was removing a pane of glass. It took him about five minutes in all, probably less. He would hammer, hammer, hammer, then pull out a pane of bone, and so on around in a circle. My whole head reverberated.

"It didn't hurt, exactly," I said when he was done. "But my inlays are definitely looser." I tried to smile.

"You see?" he said. "No problem."

"Dr. Mohs, if basal cell skin cancers like mine don't enter the blood stream—which is what I've always been told—then why all this bother? I mean, what harm would it do if, for example, you left the forehead skin cancer right there? With makeup, it would be practically invisible."

"The cancer had already invaded the bone behind your forehead," he said. "It also—unexpectedly—had gone back into your scalp. So what do you think happens if you leave an active cancer alone?"

I sighed. "I guess it continues its activity."

"Nearly always. Left alone it could have continued to grow, burrowing inward. Eventually that could mean the loss of sight in one or both eyes. It might also mean brain damage."

I felt weak, as though something had suddenly sucked the breath out of me. All these years I'd thought my type of skin cancer was only skin deep; serious only in that it could be disfiguring.

Now I thought about what might have happened had I not come to Dr. Mohs when I did . . . .

Not to be able to read, not ever again to see my children, John's face, Ted's eyes, Ellen as she grew to be a woman? And the burden I'd be to DeWitt didn't bear thinking about.

I shuddered—and thought of the other, even grimmer possibility Dr. Mohs had mentioned. Brain damage could leave me alive, yet not alive; dead, but not so dead my family could mourn, eventually cease mourning, then get on with their lives.

For the first time, I understood that this skin cancer *was really cancer.*

I went down to the lobby and had a few brief moments with myself.

What might have happened if we'd stayed in that small Iowa town instead of moving to Minnesota? I'd complained at first about living at the North Pole, but to my knowledge nobody in Iowa had ever heard of Dr. Mohs.

It was only by chance that I'd reached a doctor famous for getting out all of a cancer without damaging healthy tissue. Only through a coincidence that— Wait a minute. *Chance? Coincidence?*

I thought of a quotation from Anatole France I'd once come across:

"Chance is the pseudonym God uses when he doesn't want to sign his name."

3.

TRAUMA

I flew to Madison early on the morning of September 23 so Dr. Mohs could check me out.

"Coming along fine," he said.

"How about my nose? It seems to be all right now, but from time to time it's been crusting up and bleeding."

The crusting hadn't worried me, really, but Ellen had made me promise to ask Dr. Mohs about it. Now he pinched my nose and took a closer look. "Hmmm. Probably just a radiation-like keratosis, not really a developed cancer. I'd better biopsy it to be sure."

I was both relieved and frightened.

So he pared off a tiny piece, and sent me back to the waiting room. I sat there reading and rereading a paragraph in *Jennie, the life of Winston Churchill's mother*, while I waited for the microscopic examination results.

Rachel came into the waiting room. "Mrs. Shuck, you'd better cancel your flight. Your nose is positive."

Hoping my voice wasn't shaking as much as my hand, I called home.

"DeWitt, I'll . . . I'll be staying overnight. Dr. Mohs has found some skin cancer on my nose."

"Oh, sweetie . . . ."

"I'm calling from his office, can't tie up this phone long. Take Ellen to the Lincoln Deli for dinner. I'll get back to you tonight."

I canceled my return flight. While I was on hold to the airline, my mind flashed back to the Minneapolis dermatologist who prescribed medicinal cream for my crusting, bleeding nose.

"We don't want to touch your nose unless it's absolutely necessary," he'd told me. "The skin is tissue paper thin and your nose would need skin grafting."

Skin grafting.

I felt a panic attack building and decided to have it with the help of a martini. With a hand that was still shaking, I dialed the Ivy Inn for a reservation.

I knew they had a bar.

All day I sat in Dr. Mohs' offices. One tiny, thin slice of my nose after another was removed. Each time I waited for the microscopic evaluation; each time I prayed for a slice clear of cancer.

I tried my best to read *Jennie*, but I kept losing my place and reading the same words over and over. Though I had my head in that book all day, by evening I couldn't remember one thing about her life.

Dr. Mohs used no anesthesia other than the chemical that he painted on each tiny piece of skin that he was about to slice off and examine. The zinc chloride temporarily deadened the pain, but not all of it. Each cutting was agony.

"This hurts more than the cuttings on my forehead and chin, you know."

Dr. Mohs nodded. "Yes, the nose is more sensitive."

At one point, after he'd shaved off yet another layer, I said, "My forehead and chin are healing over nicely." Do you think what you're doing now will leave scarring?"

"There'll likely be a post-surgical defect," he said.

"Defect? Just what does that mean?"

"The cancer may not be too large," Rachel said. "The surgery might only leave a small hole in your nose."

"Only?"

"It can probably be repaired by inserting a piece of your ear, a minor surgical job."

"A piece of my *ear?*"

Rachel squeezed my upper arm, and smiled a little. "Believe me, such repairs are almost invisible," she said. "In a year or so, no one would notice anything wrong with your nose."

I didn't dare ask the question I most needed answered. There was, I realized, no earthly way anyone could know right now how much would be left of my best feature.

Finally that day was over.

I managed to get to the front entrance of University Hospital and Clinic.

"Taxi!" I called and waved. A taxi rolled over. "The Ivy Inn, please."

The driver was saying how cold and windy it was, how fast the temperature was falling—"forty degrees in the last two hours."

I kept wanting him to shut up.

Just keep control till you get to your room, Carolyn. You check in, you register, you pick up your key. And a martini-to-go. You get yourself into your room and lock the door.

"Why the nose bandage, lady?"

"Surgery."

"Oh. You break it?"

"No."

"Somebody break it for you?"

Thank God we were here.

"How much do I owe you?"

"Uh . . . two-twenty."

I handed him a five. Stumbled out. Couldn't wait for the change.

Force yourself to open that heavy door, Carolyn. On the other side of it lie room keys and martinis.

Come on. You can make it.

You have to.

Once in my room, I threw my coat on the floor, kicked off my shoes, and downed the martini. Then I took the first deep breath I'd taken since morning and sank onto the bed.

It's okay to thrash around on the bed. But don't bang your head against the wall, no matter how good you think it might feel. And whatever you do, don't cry, don't let your nose run. Rachel said to just snuffle backwards, like the little kids do.

I rolled about on the bed. Made moaning, guttural sounds. It helped a little, but what I wanted to do was to open my mouth and shriek out a scream that would shatter glass.

Dr. Mohs *told* you the nose is more sensitive than the forehead and chin.

He was right.

The physical pain had been torture, but at least it was over; and I seemed to have resources (born of recent experience?) to handle it. But my mental pain was also torture, and on that front I found myself ridiculously vulnerable. When I thought about the holes Dr. Mohs had left in my forehead and chin, it was almost more than I could bear. How much would he leave of my so recently adorable nose? I didn't know anyone who didn't have a nose.

But of course I did. Miss Margaret Murphy from Pierre, South Dakota, the woman I'd so pitied that hot sultry night last July. Was this my just dessert for patronizing a fellow sufferer? For being so secretly proud of my nose, its length and shape so perfectly suited to my face, its tip so delicately sculptured? What was happening to my best feature?

For the moment I entertained the crazy thought that maybe it wasn't happening. Maybe I had imagined it—dreamed it or dreamed it up.

I reached up carefully to touch the gauze bandage.

This was a nightmare, all right, but a *waking* bad dream. Worse, I was trapped in it—and couldn't even cry.

Nearly out of my mind, I reached out to the only person who could give me a truly informed opinion about what I was doing. I telephoned Dr. Lynch, my trusted dermatologist at the University of Minnesota.

"Carolyn," he said, "you have to let Dr. Mohs proceed. Skin cancer doesn't stand still. If this one keeps growing, you're in serious trouble."

"Okay. I'll stay. I guess I just needed to hear it."

"Then maybe you need to hear this again, too: Dr. Mohs is the foremost skin cancer surgeon in the world. He'll remove far less tissue than anyone else would have to."

I sighed. "I know you're right, Dr. Lynch."

"I'm sorry, but you really don't have any other choice."

I hung up the phone. The pain was still there, but the knowledge that losing part of my nose was inevitable somehow made it seem less nightmarish.

I'd made it through the ten hours since the biopsy showed up positive; I could surely make it through another twenty-four. Maybe by this time tomorrow evening he'd have removed all of the cancerous tissue and I'd be on my way back to Minneapolis.

Just twenty-four hours.

After two long hours of dry-eyed despair, I got my sagging self up off the sagging bed. I shook out my coat, hung it in the closet, then picked up my purse and wiped it off. Slipped my shoes back on and smoothed out my rumpled dress.

I faced myself in the oak-framed mirror above the oak dresser of that barren little hotel room and redid my lipstick and hair.

"*This*," I informed my reflection in ringing tones, "is not a tragedy."

As a child, I had lived with tragedy, knew what it was and what it could cause. Tragedy could damage or destroy human relationships, break the heart—suddenly, or slowly and inexorably so that the break couldn't heal. A minor facial disfigurement didn't even come close.

But as I looked again into that mirror, a new fear swept over me.

I'm an extrovert, always have been. I both enjoy and need closeness to other people; need to hear what's happening in their lives and to tell them what's happening in mine. And all the communication isn't verbal—with my face I'd laughed with my friends and cried with them, expressed sympathy for them and enlisted their sympathy in return.

Would they be uncomfortable, now, in my presence? Not know what to say, or where to look? With a glaring defect in the middle of my face, would I find their attention focused on that instead of on me? Would they *pity* me?

I couldn't stand that.

Looking in the mirror, I could also see that the image looking back at me didn't really match the way I saw myself.

In the mirror, I was no longer young.

But I didn't really believe that. In my imagination, I was still in my twenties or possibly my early thirties—an age at which some had called me beautiful.

I pulled up and back on the skin at either side of my neck. Not bad. I did the same with the skin in front of my ears. What an improvement.

I straightened my shoulders, and faced the mirror—squarely.

It was clear. I had to come out the other side of this skin-cancer tunnel looking better than when I entered it. No problem. Plastic surgery can accomplish miracles. Then and there I made my decision:

I would have a face lift at the same time my nose was being repaired.

I spent that evening recovering from my hours in Gethsemane over a good dinner in the hotel dining room. Chewing very carefully so as not to wiggle my nose, I thought for the first time in years about my birth defect: I'd been born prematurely and with patches of thin skin on my back, on one leg, and on my abdomen. Pink patches where the veins showed clearly through.

Dining at the Ivy Inn that night, I could still feel the shame I'd felt when I was four and my mother called my father in to point out the patches while I was having my bath. I could remember how much like a freak I'd felt when doctors touched them during a physical examination or called other doctors in to look at them or took pictures of me and my patches to send off to medical journals.

I remembered wearing culottes and stockings for the junior high picnic when all the other girls wore shorts. I was not *about* to give the others a view of the vein in my leg.

But the worst, the absolute worst, memory was of a routine physical examination at the University of Chicago when I was twenty-one. The exam took place in the morning and I had accepted a blind date with an intern that evening. As usual, a neurologist was summoned to view my patches of thin skin.

"Would you mind if I called in another doctor or two?" he asked.

It was the standard question, so I said, "Of course not . . . ."

I sat on the examining table, swinging my legs, readying my usual answers.

And almost fell off the table when a class of fifteen interns trooped through the door. They jammed the room, stood around taking notes and peering over the neurologist's shoulder while he proceeded with his tests.

I didn't dare glance at any of the interns' faces. Any one of them might be the man I was to go out with that night.

When it was finally over, I walked the five long campus blocks back to my room at International House, crying every step of the way. I felt like a freak right out of a circus side show. And I stayed in my room crying all afternoon.

I went out on the date, which was uneventful in every way. To this day, I don't know whether or not my date was in that examining room.

Looking back on it now, I suspect my thin skin areas, though unusual, weren't actually offensive to others. No child my own age ever commented on them when I was undressing in gym class, nor did my own small children ever ask about them. But their having been the subject of so much intense medical curiosity probably fostered my idea that I had a "strange" body. And though it's possible that I imagined other people's reactions, my *own* feeling about these patches was very real.

Now, twenty-nine years later, in my Madison hotel room, I tried to dial DeWitt but got no answer. I couldn't read—the thick nose bandage lifted my glasses and made the words blurry. I turned on the TV but got only local news interspersed with farm equipment ads. In the lamplight, waiting to dial DeWitt again, I thought about my family's attitude toward physical beauty.

Its importance was always played down—to the point that not once had either of my parents ever told me I was pretty. Good looks were a superficial attribute, in no way comparable to integrity, kindness, or the desire to leave the world better for having been in it.

I did not disagree with this lofty view, but as a teenager and then as a young woman I was delighted to get compliments from young men. It was reassuring to know that though I was afflicted with hidden patches of thin skin, the part of me that went unclothed was considered attractive.

There was one young man who had been a good friend for seven years and a would-be fiancé for the three years after that. Before falling for me, he'd always dated very pretty girls—would he change his opinion or his feelings if I told him about my patches? After all, even Queen Victoria couldn't keep her clothes on at all times after she married.

"I have these pale pink patches of skin on my leg and back," I said one night when he again brought up the subject of marriage. "Would this affect your feeling for me after we married?"

He looked puzzled, but he took a few seconds to think. "No," he said, finally, "it won't make any difference at all."

Somehow, as soon as he said it, I knew I could believe him.

And so, when he said, "You're beautiful, Carolyn," I believed that too.

And the next time DeWitt Shuck brought up the subject of marriage, I said, "Yes."

Twenty-nine years later, alone in a hotel room, I dialed my husband for a third time. Still no answer. What was taking them so long? They couldn't very well get a five-course meal in a delicatessen.

I settled back to wait some more and remember some more.

Two decades ago, a business appointment in Mexico City made it convenient for us to plan spending part of our honeymoon in that city and part of it on the beach in Acapulco. *On the beach in a bathing suit?* My thin skin patches would be on display to the world. And to DeWitt.

I spent months searching, searching the stores for a becoming swimsuit before I finally found a figure-flattering orchid number. Years later I was to learn that orchid is the only color DeWitt truly detests. But at the moment I first appeared in the suit, I was conscious only of my skin patches.

DeWitt didn't seem to notice them, so I didn't mention my distress. But as things turned out, at least a dozen people from Keokuk—that small Iowa town where I was soon to arrive as a bride—had also decided to vacation in Acapulco that February. And they, like us, spent most mornings and afternoons on the beach.

At first I felt as though I'd been forced to parade nude down Keokuk's main street. But thrown in to sink or swim on our honeymoon, I swam. And to make sure I wouldn't drown, I swam with all my might, doing my best to be charming, loving, and lovable. I kept telling myself I'd been put on this earth for a purpose: that love and good were meant to flow through my flawed body to others as easily and as much as through a perfect body.

It worked. For many years we repeatedly joined the same couples in Acapulco for winter beach holidays, and these old beach buddies are still among our closest friends. I doubt that DeWitt found anything about my bathing-suited appearance off-putting other than my suit's orchid color, and I suspect that the Iowans never paid much—if any—attention to my supposed defects.

Jane, for instance, was gorgeous, witty, flawlessly groomed; her husband Bob was suave and smooth, a successful businessman who enjoyed driving fancy sports cars. During a month in Acapulco with the two of them, DeWitt was recuperating from the mumps and had to go to bed early every evening—leaving Jane, Bob, and me to stay up until all hours, enjoying tequila and one another.

"If I have to make a ten-minute report at the hospital auxiliary meeting,"

Jane said on one of these occasions, "it scares me so much I have diarrhea for a week." Over the years she confessed to many other feelings of inadequacy in areas where I had great confidence.

Bob turned out to have a father who'd driven a taxi in the same small town where Bob was now president of a nationally known company. "Because I never went to college," he said on one Acapulco evening, "I often feel inferior to the men who rank under me. It bugs me all the time."

Now I knew why Bob always had to drive the latest sports car, why Jane never had a chipped finger nail. Neither Bob nor Jane or any of the others cared what I looked like; they only cared how I thought *they* looked.

All the time I'd been so busy hiding my legs and back, these apparently self-assured people had their own thin-skinned areas they were hiding. Bob and Jane needed acceptance and under-standing, just as I did—along with just about everyone else I'd ever come to know well.

I reached for the phone again, then stopped. Didn't the lesson I'd learned on the beaches of Acapulco so long ago still apply? To whatever extent the cancer left my nose disfigured, the people I encountered would be far more concerned with how they appeared to me than how I appeared to them.

I called home again. Still no answer. It must be about ten o'clock, I thought, but I checked my watch. Only eight-fifteen?

Apparently my memories and the philosophizing they produced had occupied less than an hour.

The next time I tried, DeWitt answered.

"How are you getting along?" DeWitt asked.

I wanted to pour out all my fears to him but knew his aversion to illness would stop me from doing anything of the kind.

"Well, okay, I guess. Really, I'm fine. And certainly feeling better than I was a few hours ago. Dr. Mohs will probably finish tomorrow."

"So what did you have for dinner?" Ellen asked. Without waiting for my reply, she continued "I had fried chicken, corn on the cob, mashed potatoes with yummy gravy, carrot salad, rootbeer, chocolate cake, and peppermint ice cream, and we got some maca-roons and sugar donuts at the bakery counter."

They *had* managed a seven course dinner in a delicatessen.

"When does your flight arrive?" DeWitt asked me.

"I'll call you when I've made a reservation and give you the flight number."

But I didn't make it home the next evening, or the evening after that. For six more days Dr. Mohs had to keep paring away skin from my nose, cutting away thin slice after thin slice, layer after layer. All of them were proving cancerous.

Would I have any nose left?

I had to push myself into his offices each day, telling myself I'd made it through the last twenty-four hours, surely I could get through just one more twenty-four hour span. But the twenty-four hour spans were getting longer.

Looking down at me from Dr. Mohs' office wall was the picture of a broadly smiling baby, captioned: SMILE.

"I like your baby picture, but the caption could use some editing," I said.

"How's that?"

"It should read: SMILE—Dr. Mohs is going to leave some of you."

"I'll change it tomorrow."

As things progressed, and cutting followed cutting, Rachel stopped squeezing my arm or telling me that my nose would easily be patched with a piece of my ear. She seemed to be affixing those dressings on my nose a bit more firmly, quickly, even a little more painfully. It was as though her hands were delivering messages like: "There now. That's not so bad. Get going."

It was the same manner I'd affected when my small children weren't just scratched up, but badly hurt, hoping they'd be less frightened if I seemed authoritative and unconcerned. Maybe Rachel was hoping I'd never suspect she knew the extent of the cancer, unexpectedly much deeper than originally anticipated and involving the tip and cartilage of the nose.

"All right, you," she said, "now go out in the waiting room and cheer up those other patients."

I did, using all the strength I could muster. But Rachel didn't fool me, not for a minute. Try as she might to look unconcerned, I felt her overwhelming empathy.

DeWitt arrived in Madison on the fourth harrowing day. For all my assurances on the telephone—"I'm fine, really"—he'd called Dr. Mohs, then decided to come.

The emotional pain and physical anguish I'd been going through were pretty awful, but clearly I was handling the ordeal. So why in the world should DeWitt have to suffer through it too? And didn't I have good reason to know that sometimes you have to be braver if you're by yourself?

Although I'd told him there was really no need for him to come, the minutes dragged by on the day he was to arrive. When he finally walked into my room at the Ivy Inn, it was as though the Messiah had appeared.

How I wanted to cry with sheer joy as he enveloped me in his arms—so very, very gently—for a long, comforting moment. Instead, I had to grit my teeth lest my nose run or bleed, or both.

I leaned back so I could look into his face.

"I need a big hug." I said.

"I'm afraid I'll hurt you, sweetie."

"You won't. Please."

Turning his head to keep from bumping my nose, he gingerly embraced me, then stepped back.

"Remember how weak you were when you came home from Madison the first time? Well, Barbara Johnson called when she heard you were here and told me to go out and get a blender so I can fix you this drink." He pulled a small scrap of paper from his pocket with a recipe pencilled on it. "I'll go get this stuff before the stores close."

The chemicals used in the removal had left me with no appetite and additional cutting made chewing impossible. I *was* getting woozy.

Soon DeWitt had permission to use the Ivy Inn kitchen to make the blender concoction and store his ingredients. The drink made me feel much stronger. The next day I went from patient to patient in Dr. Mohs' waiting room, selling the idea that each and every one of them would benefit from a miracle drink made of milk, powdered milk, eggs, and frozen orange concentrate.

I could also have told each one something far more important: send for a loved one. No one should go through hell alone.

Simply by being there, DeWitt lifted my spirits no end. Knowing he'd come because he wanted to and not because I'd summoned him helped even more. I had to get through six extremely painful hours a day, but there were also some hours each day free of pain.

During these pain-free hours, DeWitt and I shared observations about the other patients, imagining their lives in the outside world. We smiled together over Ellen's homesickness for camp now that she was back in school in Minneapolis. We enjoyed John's description of a new pal at Amherst. We wondered if we'd ever have a letter from Ted. And, as always, we talked of what was happening in DeWitt's business.

The last thing on my mind during all of this was how I looked. Everyone in Dr. Mohs' office was in the same boat, and the Ivy Inn housed several guests who wore his tell-tale bandaging.

By noon on Saturday he was done. All the malignancies in the skin and cartilage were gone. When I heard him say, "We're through, Mrs. Shuck,"

I stood up, then fell into Rachel's arms with relief. *No more cutting.*

"You're as beautiful as ever, except for your nose," Dr. Mohs said.

"And a plastic surgeon can fix that."

I looked in the mirror over the sink in his office.

Judas.

My whole face was swollen and distorted, and there at its center—I turned away.

As beautiful as ever!

"When can I get it rebuilt?"

"Not for six months."

"Six months? Why in the world do I have to wait six months? I'm perfectly healthy and this will heal up long before that. Remember how quickly my forehead and chin healed?"

"I'll want to check your nose and your whole face carefully over the next six months. We want to be sure no new cancers sprout up. I don't want any future trouble covered up by premature reconstruction."

So. This was what I'd look like, for half a year. I faced the mirror, and this time didn't turn away.

There was a large oblong hole through the right side of my nose about the size of my thumbnail, and a smaller hole through the left side. A good deal of the tip was also gone.

Much of my nose had simply disappeared.

4.

LIFE RESUMES

My reentry to normal life after the nose surgery was easier than after Dr. Mohs had worked on my forehead and chin. True, the physical and emotional trauma had been greater but this time I had the blender concoction and a husband to keep up my strength. By now I was an old hand at dousing my wounds with mercurochrome, and I also had DeWitt's help to get me home, a real Godsend.

This time, coming home from Madison meant coming home to Ellen, who rushed up with a hearty hug before I was all the way inside the door.

"Gosh, I'm glad you're back. I hope you're not mad at me for saying Dr. Mohs should check your nose."

I shook my fist at her. "You and your big mouth. Seriously, Ellen, I'll never be able to thank you enough. If you hadn't reminded me, I might not have mentioned it."

"Does it hurt?"

"Not now."

"I'm never going out in the sun again."

"Your skin isn't like mine, it's like your Dad's. He can play golf all day and his face never burns. What's going on at school?"

"Well, you won't believe this, but Mrs. Cole told us she really used to believe that football players actually had those humongous shoulders. She didn't know they wore pads. Did Dr. Mohs hurt you a lot?"

So much for changing the subject.

"As little as possible, but yes, it hurt. Anyway, it's all over now. In six months I can get it fixed by a plastic surgeon. They'll knock me out so it won't hurt while they're working."

She gave me another hug—tight enough to make me wonder if my now eleven-year-old daughter planned to try out for the football team.

"That's good," she said. "I don't want you to hurt."

In a few days I felt as though I were weeks away from the nose surgery. My life had resumed its busy pace, which helped. And I used up plenty of energy devising ingenious solutions to problems the current state of my nose created.

One of my first challenges was devising a painless way to read. It hurt to have my reading glasses rest on the nose bandage, so I wound tape around their bridge, leaving a two-inch tail that I stuck to my forehead. With my glasses hanging just above the bandage, I could still see—and without any pressure on my nose.

Toward the end of my second week at home, nose still in a white bandage, I headed out for Dayton's Department Store—eight minutes from my garage to theirs—and shopped for an hour with efficiency and no self-consciousness whatsoever.

I saw my good friend Mary Sue Reed looking at sweaters in the next department over—and then, when I waved, looking at me. The shock on her face was replaced almost immediately by a smile as she started walking up to me.

I took hold of her arms and smiled back.

"Mary Sue, didn't you notice something was just a little different?"

"What happened?"

"I had a skin cancer operation, but in six months I can have it repaired. How are things with the Tuesday golfers?"

"I was going to ask if you'd be chairman this year."

"Sure. Do we meet this coming Tuesday?"

"Yes. Probably one of the last golf days of the season."

"It'll be great to be back. Sign me up to play with someone, will you?

"I've got to go—Ellen will be home at four, ready to beat me at hearts."

That hadn't been hard at all. Of course, all Mary could see was a bandage . . . .

I pushed the button on the elevator to the parking ramp. A car stopped, already carrying enough people so that I had to back into it. The closing doors barely missed my face. I recoiled, touched the nose bandage, and said, "Oh! I wouldn't want it to happen *again.*"

Horrified looks—and hushed silence—greeted this comment. Three floors later I got off, managing not to laugh until I was in my car. I could just imagine the dinner table conversation of my fellow passengers in a few hours:

"Don't ever stand too close to an elevator door, son. I saw a woman today who actually . . ."

I'm not completely sure where I got the idea that repairing my nose would be a simple process. But it was probably when Dr. Mohs said ". . . and a plastic surgeon can fix that."

My nose deformity would be only temporary, like a fender dent you had to wait six months to have pounded out and repainted. I would wait out the winter of 1970, then be good-as-new lovely in the spring of '71.

Ten days after coming home, I flew back to Madison for Dr. Mohs to remove the outer crust. This mission accomplished, I looked into the mirror, turning from side to side as I tried to get an impression of what my nose looked like without a crust.

"Maybe this is my one big chance to set a trend," I said. "Not nose rings, but nose jewels. A huge emerald to fill the biggest hole, an almost-huge diamond for the smaller one."

"There you go," Dr. Mohs said. "You could become a Hindu."

Rachel took hold of my shoulder and turned me toward the door.

"Go across the street to the drug store and get some flesh-colored Micropore tape. It'll cover your nose defects wonderfully until you have plastic surgery."

The drugstore carried more flesh-colored Micropore tape than any other variety—obviously the store's proximity to Dr. Mohs' office created a steady flow of customers. Micropore came in rolls of different widths, like Scotch Tape, and was made by the same manufacturer. Beige-pink, tissue-paper thin, and translucent, it was lightweight and unobtrusive—not at all like adhesive tape.

I bought a roll, quickly tore off a piece, and stuck it on the back of my hand. It was hardly visible, taking on the color of my skin.

At home, I carefully cut a pattern the exact size and shape to cover my nose holes. Then, using the pattern, I cut dozens of nose covers from a roll of inch-wide tape and pasted them on foil-covered shirt cardboards. In two seconds I could peel one off and smooth it over what was left of my nose. It could be removed just as easily.

Many times I silently thanked the stranger who'd invented the tape. Without it, life would have been far more daunting and difficult. Adhesive tape or a Band-Aid would've been far more conspicuous, and repeated use of either would have aggravated my tender nose skin.

But as good as it was, Micropore tape couldn't actually replace the missing skin. Never before had I been aware of how the nose warms the air as it's inhaled. That winter seemed especially frigid, even for Minnesota.

"I'd give anything for a stick-on mink nose muff," I once said to DeWitt.

He nodded. "I'll bet you would."

The Micropore tape camouflaged things well enough that I felt I looked quite presentable, especially from a distance. There was no grotesque deformity. The rest of my face looked as it always had. My forehead and chin had healed over nicely.

I'd always been amazed by women who could sit at a dressing table for seemingly endless hours applying foundation, rouge, gluing on false eyelashes, and putting on eye liner and mascara. Once I'd tried to "do" my eyes, but after three minutes the project became so tedious I abandoned it. I didn't even own a hand mirror to look at the sides or back of my hair. In its absence, I was unaware of how my profile had changed.

Trying on dresses in a fitting room with three-way mirrors, I was shocked to see my profile resembled Peter Rabbit's. We both had snubbed off noses. Instead of buying a hand mirror, I decided to avoid three-way mirrors until my normal profile was restored.

I knew my nose wasn't a problem that would go away if I ignored it, but I also knew that if I disregarded it, other people probably would too.

My days were active. I managed a household that could on a day's notice become a bed-and-breakfast, with dinner thrown in. John and Ted were in college, but the extended vacations they spent with us often involved housing and feeding their buddies as well. Ellen's hobbies and friends were many, varied, and constantly changing, but her plans usually seemed to include me as a chauffeur.

I was also putting a great deal of energy that year into starting a women's clinic in the poorest section of Minneapolis. Women who rarely saw a doctor between childbirths began coming in every six months for breast exams, pap smears, and blood pressure checks as well as instruction in birth control. I'd started a similar clinic when we lived in Iowa and knew the good it could do.

In addition, DeWitt and I led an active social life. Some involved DeWitt's business, but most was for sheer enjoyment. My days were full, some hectic. And through it all, my nose didn't seem to bother friends or acquaintances much at all.

During this period I was invited to join a sewing club.

"Terrific," I said. "I could bring my mending."

"Oh no. We don't sew."

Instead they met in each other's homes for elaborate luncheons. All the members except myself had become friends at an exclusive private school and had remained close for over forty years. As a newly arrived outsider—and an outsider with a defective nose at that—I appreciated being taken in by "Old Minneapolis" society.

On Fridays I played bridge with three friends. We were all new to Minneapolis, and I never had more fun than with these three women. Liza was a New Englander who referred to her husband as the Boss, and to her rich next door neighbors who claimed poverty as "the Weez-po's."

My friendship with Peg went back to Keokuk, where we goaded each other into highly creative escapades we never talked about in front of children, husbands, or friends. Norma was a lapsed southerner, who liked to say, "I never tell my age, no one would believe me that young." Norma was a superb bridge player; unfortunately for her, bridge to the rest of us, was only something to do with our hands while we talked.

Norma had said one Friday that a mutual acquaintance who knew about the bridge group had asked her what I was going to do about my . . . problem.

"So how did you answer?"

"I told her, 'We don't sit around and discuss Carolyn's nose, you know.' "

Undoubtedly this woman was expressing concern out of kindness. But, what an inane way of thinking. Did she also worry about whether or not a pregnant woman would have her baby? After all, my nose would be fixed up after six months.

"I can imagine how you must feel," John said when he came home at Christmas. "I've always been self-conscious about a few acne scars."

"But it's only temporary. There are only three months left to go in my six-month waiting period. By your spring break, it'll be fixed. The truth is, John, *I'm* not self-conscious about it, so don't you worry about it."

"Sure, mom. Bet you can't wait until spring, can you?"

Ted arrived from Oregon with hugs and concern.

"I love you, Mom. I'm really sorry Dr. Mohs had to do so much more work on your face. Hope it wasn't too painful."

"You mean all that cutting was supposed to *hurt?*" I looked at his face and saw he didn't find my pain an appropriate topic for humor. "It could have been worse. Can't you see how well my forehead and chin have healed? Since early September?"

"They really have."

After their initial outpouring of sympathy, the children accepted my reassurances. Their friends filled the house as usual, and they seemed as unaware of the way I looked as did John, Ted, and Ellen. Essentially, I think, their reactions mirrored my own: the disfigurement was temporary, more an inconvenience than anything else.

John would say, "Mom, pull down the tape a little on the right side of your nose; it isn't quite covering," in the same tone of voice he might use to say, "Mom, your slip's showing."

Oddly enough, I never really worried about what DeWitt thought. For all my self-consciousness about my thin-skin patches, I had not a qualm about how he might react to a far more serious defect. After twenty years of living with him, I knew he appreciated beauty but also saw it for what it is, a superficial trait. I also knew nothing superficial would ever come between us.

I didn't worry about what DeWitt thought, and DeWitt didn't share any worries he had on my behalf. It's not that he couldn't feel compassion but that he couldn't express it—especially where illness was concerned.

"I'm worried about Bob," he'd say. "His double vision seems to be getting worse." And then later, "Has Jean said anything to you about Bob? How's he doing?"

"Why don't you ask him?"

I knew, of course, that the last thing DeWitt would do is say anything to *Bob*. Did he think mentioning Bob's double vision would be an invasion of privacy? Did he think if he *didn't* say anything it would just go away?

For certain people—and DeWitt for whatever reason was certainly among them—it's so hard to *accept* illness that talking about it is practically impossible. In my experience a great many men are like DeWitt, and even those who can accept illness or disability may very well not be able to put their concern into words.

I understood all of this. But it's also hard to live in the same house with the person you love without talking about the subject that's most on your mind.

So when I said, "I do look a bit odd with this pared-down nose, don't I?"

And he said, "Oh, that's ridiculous . . . ."

I knew he thought I did look odd, but didn't find that important in the least.

I have to say, there were times when his eyes looked a little watery. If he didn't have a cold, I might start wondering: Are those *tears* I'm seeing?

Surely not. The nose surgery hadn't been unbearable, and in any case I had borne it. All I needed now was a simple nose repair, during which the doctors would put me to sleep.

I wouldn't even have to help them do the operation.

That fall and winter, I searched magazines for pictures of gorgeous noses, clipping ones I especially liked and putting them in a folder.

When I worried that other people's eyes would be drawn to my defective nose instead of to me, I hadn't realized my own eyes would be drawn to noses. I'd have to force my eyes away so I could concentrate on what the nose owner was saying.

At one point, while studying the nose of a Minneapolis friend, I managed to listen long enough for her to tell me about a plastic surgeon who'd taken care of her elderly mother.

"He removed a skin cancer on her cheek by taking it from the inside of her mouth," she said, "That way, it didn't show."

Clearly an ingenious surgeon.

I got his name and made an appointment to see him, and sat waiting with Ellen outside his office door until my name was called.

"Okay, Mrs. Shuck," the doctor said. "Let's see what we have to work with."

I quickly removed the Micropore tape from my nose.

"What in *God's name* have they been *doing* to you?"

"A . . . a doctor—Dr. Mohs, in Madison, Wisconsin—removed skin cancer from my nose."

"Good God." He threw up his hands. "I've never seen such a thing in my life! I can't do anything with *that.*"

I felt deeply shamed, as though he'd found evidence beneath the Micropore of my having taken a knife and butchered my best feature.

I left his office as fast as I could, concentrated on concealing my anguish from Ellen, and drove straight home. This doctor had never seen nose wounds like mine, much less tried to repair them. Did this mean *no* plastic surgeon could repair my nose? Sick at heart, I was also sick to my stomach.

"Mom, is something wrong?" Ellen asked me that evening. "You didn't eat a thing for dinner—and you never told me what the doctor said—what went on this afternoon, anyway?"

"He looked at my nose . . . ."

"And?"

"And he was . . . horrified. He said he wouldn't even attempt to repair it. It was pretty scary, but I'll be fine, I don't . . . ."

"Mom, didn't you tell me how Dr. Mohs' office is always crowded with patients from all over the country?"

"Yes."

"Well, you were the only patient in that waiting room this afternoon. If I were you, I'd believe what Dr. Mohs told me."

I grinned, kissed her goodnight—and wondered just who was the child in this scenario.

I wouldn't let my mind so much as touch on the consultation with the plastic surgeon. Nor did I mention the incident to anyone. I was not going to allow any doubt in anyone's mind—including mine—that my nose would be successfully repaired after six months.

And in the meantime, I kept dealing with the disfigurement in my own way.

I went to Oklahoma to transact some business with a lawyer I'd known since childhood.

"What happened to you?" he asked right off.

"Syphilis," I said.

Another lawyer came into his office.

"Harold," my friend said with no change of expression, "this is Carolyn Shuck. She's had syphilis."

I loved the way he handled our meeting. It showed nothing had really changed.

Then there was the woman who said, "Aren't you glad this happened at your age?"

Inwardly, I'd smiled. I *was* fortunate to get this cancer while I was still young enough to heal easily.

"After all," she said, "For a *young* person, being disfigured could cause a real nervous breakdown."

I assumed she meant one lasting more than two hours.

At night I'd still dream from time to time about parts of my nose being sliced off. I'd awaken—my hand flying up to my face—expecting the wonderful relief you feel when you realize what you've dreamed isn't real, didn't happen.

But that relief could never come. The nightmare, although I was learning to deal more and more with it, was still very real.

5.

LONG, LONG AGO

It was 1924, and oh, what fun it was to sit on the basement stairs on a Sunday morning with my older sister, Marjorie. Our father polished our shoes for Sunday School as we held up each foot in turn. Our shoes were white, buttoned up the sides, and had black patent toes and heels.

Our hair had been washed and rolled up in rag curlers the night before. Now it had been brushed out into soft blonde curls.

We'd had our oatmeal, and soon we'd be out in the front yard where our father would take our picture by the big oak tree whose trunk was so huge they'd had to build the sidewalk around it in a semi-circle.

Our black straw hats were wide-brimmed with long black streamers. Marjorie was two years older than I but we were always dressed alike. Sometimes we were mistaken for twins.

My father would take our pictures with his Kodak. It was a magical contraption. An accordion-pleated protrusion held a big glass eye and in it we could see the birdie if we looked closely as he told us to smile.

My mother would fix a roast. She put it in the oven with the potatoes, and we ate it just as soon as we came home from Sunday School and church. The homemade ice cream was in the crank-type freezer in the basement with the rock salt and rag rugs piled around to keep it cool.

I liked sitting in church with my father. He drew one entertaining picture after another, mostly dogs and horses. And if I got sleepy, my mother would take me onto her lap for a short nap. Her lap was so soft, so warm. When I awoke, I could look up into her lovely face and into her luminous, smiling blue eyes.

Once in a while my mother's two sisters came for an extended visit. After graduating from the University of Nebraska, they'd chosen to teach in South India rather than South Omaha. They'd become missionaries and ran a school for famine orphans.

When they visited, our lifestyle did change a little. The playing cards were put away and devotions were read three times a day, before meals. But things didn't dull down; they picked up.

The devotions consisted of scripture readings accompanied by sermonettes, exciting because my aunts' true adventure stories were interwoven with the message.

For instance, while learning about trust, I found out that if a snake should crawl beneath your nightgown and down your back while you were trying to get some sleep on a hot night, you were to lie perfectly still and try not to breathe until that snake went away.

But aside from important lessons in such practical matters, a strong impression came through that if you were like the Good Samaritan and followed the teachings of Jesus, your life was bound to be happy.

There was a solid feeling that everything was going to be just dandy, because there was a God who would always love you. The concept became as firmly planted in my mind as the idea that every morning it would become light, and every evening night would fall.

How exciting it was to teeter around the low windowsills of our breakfast room with Marjorie, both of us trying to keep our balance while walking precariously on those narrow sills. And we had great fun playing dolls in our nursery.

The only pain Marjorie ever caused me, that I can remember, was when she went out to play, just one time, before I woke up from my nap. There I was, awake, and she was gone.

I remember a day when Marjorie wouldn't make a funny face back at me. Mother explained that Marjorie didn't feel well.

Or that other day, after her tonsillectomy, when they put a white kitchen chair behind her bed pillow so that she could sit up and get her breath.

Then came another day, more terrible than any other, when they told me Marjorie had gone to be with Louise, my twin sister, who had died four years earlier at the age of two weeks.

I couldn't believe Marjorie would leave me to be with Louise.

"You're fooling me," I said.

But later, when I carried in Marjorie's doll, my father took it from my arms.

"You're never to play with any of Marjorie's toys."

Then I did believe them.

My world was suddenly not the same. Death had torn away my favorite playmate. Marjorie would never again be there when I woke up from my nap.

Some nights I hoped she could look down at me through a star.

We still made ice cream in the crank-type freezer, my mother still rolled my hair up in rag curlers every night, my father still polished up my shoes every Sunday morning as I sat alone on the basement steps. But the house was seldom filled with the sunshine of laughter and carefree fun. More often than not it was filled with a leaden, oppressive feeling.

I believe that Marjorie's death put a devastating strain on my parents' marriage. Year by year, their relationship deteriorated from one of love and harmony to one filled with hurt. But in those days, even people who could severely hurt each other didn't separate. My parents stayed together.

Two strong assets helped them: they had intellectual camaraderie, occasionally enjoying stimulating arguments over books and politics; and each had a superb sense of humor coupled with an unbeatable sense of the ridiculous. There were times when they were joined together in a pressure-relieving laugh over an inescapably funny episode. It may have been part of the glue that made them stick together.

Friends told me my mother wasn't ever quite the same after Marjorie died. Still good company, never bitter, but she was never able to be quite so young at heart again.

My father was never the same again at all. He kept all of Marjorie's toys and clothing in a huge cedar chest. It was not to be opened or removed from our house, ever.

And it didn't help that just after he lost Marjorie, my father's business failed. As years went by he became more embittered, easily enraged, and sometimes cruel.

There are ways of beating one's wife without touching her; as he grew older, my father became skilled in some of these ways. As a trapped observer of his hideous verbal abuse of my mother, I felt tortured and helpless. These were not the fair fights that clear the air in a normal marriage. They could become wild, threatening storms in which I felt my mother would surely perish.

Why my mother didn't leave, I couldn't understand. Maybe she couldn't abandon the man my father had once been. Perhaps she realized then, as I do now, that my father was both a terrible and a wonderful man.

At the time, I only knew that I longed to escape.

I think that such an existence did provide benefits. It gave me perspective. For the rest of my life, thorns in the flesh would remain thorns, they would not become sabers.

And it made me unconsciously determined, even as a child, never to be unhappy again.

My childhood was not filled only with sadness. Not by a long shot, it wasn't. My parents were constant in their love for me, my aunts visited us often, and I discovered there was an escape from those threatening storms that could so unexpectedly descend to make my home unbearable. My neighborhood became a paradise; an escape to an exciting, exhilarating, fun-packed outside world.

For a time my father had enjoyed great success as an oil broker. My parents built a large home in Tulsa; but as oil deals often do, one after another fell through. Shortly before Marjorie died, we had moved to a small house in a modest neighborhood where one could count thirty-seven kids on the block. It was a step down for my parents, but what a lucky step up it was for me. I had thirty-seven new playmates. I needed them once Marjorie was gone.

Betty Wilcox and I became cronies. She had spirit and was loaded with good ideas. It was hard to keep up with her as she jumped from a garage roof, shinnied down a water pipe, climbed up into a catalpa tree. But, oh, the delight of playing out doors with her and the others on a mild spring evening.

My parents' money was suddenly gone, but even in our new, modest neighborhood each house had behind it a single-car garage attached to which there was a servant's quarters to house the "help"—the employees who did the scrubbing, laundry, and cooking for these young families.

Every day Betty and I stole into these quarters and examined each possession. There were long dangling rhinestone earrings to be tried on, castoff evening shoes to be clumped around in, red satin blouses to be held up while one admired oneself in small, scarred, oval dressing table mirrors.

I remember those dark little rooms, the heavy old draperies closed against the Oklahoma heat, the musty smell of the bottle-green mohair sofas, the tables covered with worn maroon velvet cloths that dropped to the floor. Piles of already over-used clothing were stacked on furniture or in corners. A whole family might occupy a room only ten by twelve feet. They didn't at all seem dreary to me. They were mysterious dens, comfy and cozy. Perhaps that was because I knew most of the occupants well, and they were comfy, cozy people themselves.

On the hottest summer afternoons we would retire to Betty's front porch where we sat at a miniature table and sipped her mother's perfume from tiny tea cups. I didn't really like the taste, but I wasn't about to chicken out on Betty. Today after dinner, when the best brandy is served, I'm back with Betty on that front porch, having a touch of Bellodgia, a sip of My Sin.

Many times I've wondered why her mother never missed that perfume.

But there was a generous assortment of bottles on her mother's dressing table because her father was on a winning streak. The bottles might not be there tomorrow, but they were there today.

Today. That was the day that was lived to the fullest in my extended neighborhood family.

Why would anyone worry about the dry hole of yesterday? Why worry about tomorrow? Today was to be celebrated, and celebrate we did.

When I left Oklahoma and went away to Carleton College in Minnesota, the greatest shock I suffered was my exposure to people who were intensely serious. They seemed to be going through life with teeth clenched, shoulders braced against imaginary gales. Some not only cried over spilt milk, but insisted on swimming in it. From time to time, though, I met a blithe spirit with an appreciation of the comical, and we became fast friends.

Temperament and resiliency are somewhat inborn, but I think there were some special reasons why my days were much the same as they had been when I was a child after a lot of my nose was removed. One was my grandmother.

In 1889, when my mother was only two, her father died. My grandmother was left with nine children and a cash income of twenty dollars a month. It goes without saying that things were austere in my grandmother's household as far as material things were concerned. But she spent her wisdom, love, and humor with abandon.

Grandmother's formula for bringing up children was simple: give them love and a lot of freedom. Lack of money probably furnished necessary discipline.

When my mother was three, she climbed up onto the kitchen cupboard and helped herself to handfuls of sugar cubes.

"Mabel, you eat all the sugar cubes you want," my grandmother said.

My mother continued to stuff herself. The sugar cubes got sweeter and sweeter, but the more she ate, the sicker she felt. She never got into the sugar cubes again.

Her formula worked. All her children became well-educated, productive, interesting people.

From both my parents I learned to look on the brighter side of things. My father, for instance, held many jobs while he worked his way through the University of Nebraska, getting up at four every morning to fire furnaces, and kept busy long into the night. He also sent money home to help support his family. Unable to buy an overcoat, on cold days he stuffed newspapers under his jacket as insulation. Yet he became president of his senior class. When he recounted his college days to me, his reminiscences weren't colored with self-pity; rather they were entertaining stories of exciting days.

My mother taught eight grades in a one-room country school to earn money to enter the University of Nebraska. She boarded with a farmer's family and rode horseback to and from her work. Such a jouncing ride couldn't have been easy, as she was never robust.

Her stories about teaching the one-room school never dwelt on the hardship of commuting by horseback in Nebraska's winter storms, the difficulty of building the schoolhouse fire, or the task of cleaning the outhouse on a sub-zero morning. Rather, I remember stories of Oscar, still a grammar school student at twenty, who had a crush on his younger teacher. To her dismay, he insisted on escorting her to and from school on his own horse. And when she admonished her pupils to keep the outhouse more tidy, he'd stood up in class to say, "Miss Nelson, I just want you to know it wasn't me."

My father was still in the oil business, although on a reduced scale. It often took my father away from home, so I spent a lot of time with my mother. And I learned to admire and covet her boundless aplomb. Shopping in downtown Tulsa, we had stopped to examine the contents of a department store window, when the elastic in her underpants gave way. Suddenly they were around her ankles on the sidewalk. I was mortified and wanted to hide from the other shoppers. But mother simply stepped out of her unmentionables and dropped them into her closed but unstrapped umbrella. Unfazed, she continued to peruse the display.

In 1927 my father's oil ventures forced him to spend three boiling summer months in Eldorado, Arkansas. Mother rented our Tulsa home and took me with her to Juneau, Alaska. That year, people were permitted to climb freely about on the Mendenhall glacier. Peering down into deep blue ice crevasses, I shook with fright. But glacier climbing fascinated my mother.

On a boat trip, mother wanted the guides to take her picture as she stood on an iceberg. They protested it wouldn't be safe, since the iceberg could tip over. Today we have a picture of my mother standing on an iceberg, smiling.

Later, when she couldn't climb around on glaciers and icebergs, she was still investigative, mentally active, and busy. She read widely, built and decorated a new house, gardened, designed clothes and had them made.

In 1940, my father gave her the proceeds from the sale of a small bungalow. It was his best investment. Mother spent several hours a day researching and analyzing the balance sheets of corporations. She was so successful in the stock market, Bernard Baruch would have paid her for lessons.

As a parent, she was a lot like her own mother, giving me a lot of love and a lot of freedom. When she was going through a bad period in her life, and would like to have kept me nearby, she nevertheless sent me to a school far from home. It took courage, but she got out of my way so I could get a quality education.

My mother never told me I was pretty; nor did she tell me I was smart. It's a good thing, because she did give me a compliment once, and that compliment got me into all sorts of jams.

"Carolyn, you can do anything in the world, if you just put your mind to it."

I took that compliment so to heart that on my second job, I thought I knew how to run the place. I answered the mail and filed it away without showing it to my boss.

Maybe mother was short on the compliments, but from her own experience, she knew you have to build your own confidence and strength.

For the last twenty years of her life my mother had osteoporosis and wore a back brace at all times. She also had severe angina and popped nitroglycerine pills the way a candy addict might down gum drops. On her visits, DeWitt and I ignored her physical problems because she seemed to ignore them.

"I've heard osteoporosis is painful, but you don't seem to have any pain," I once said to her.

"I'm in constant pain, but I decided years ago never to become an invalid."

She died of a heart attack just before she was eighty.

Her daily journal lay on her desk. I read her last entry:

> Planted iris bulbs. Cleaned downstairs hall linen closet.
>
> Read to page 234 in *The Eighth Day*. May get oxygen tent. To Effie's for delicious luncheon: crab louie, avocado salad, her marvelous homemade rolls with plum jam, and chocolate roll. General Motors up 2-3/8.

"May get oxygen tent" was wedged in, almost as an afterthought, among all the other things she'd found so interesting that day. "The world is so full of a number of things, I'm sure we should all be as happy as kings," she had quoted to me, over and over.

That's what life was for my mother: much too full of a number of interesting things for her to waste time or thought on ailments that couldn't be rectified. I'd like to think that I'm a little like my mother—that the apple didn't fall too far from the tree.

Even after Marjorie died, when I spent time alone with my father it could be a lot of fun. Many things my father contributed to my life enriched it. He relished life, savoring every moment. When a thunderstorm approached, he didn't run into the house and turn off the electricity. He'd call me out to watch it with him. His appreciation of the storm's wonder was contagious, and today I love thunderstorms too.

Unlike a number of people educated as engineers, my father had very wide interests. He had an avid preoccupation with history, and an intense curiosity about everything else on the face of the earth. His curiosity about how things worked passed on to me.

I once combined my mother's compliment with my father's insatiable curiosity. As I tried to repair an ancient Minnesota furnace, lightning bolts split the nylon handle of my screwdriver. I was all but electrocuted.

And he teased me. There was no hostility, only the notion that I was not only lovable, but comical. It wasn't long before I, too, realized I was sometimes comical. He taught me to laugh at myself.

Except for a few lean years, my father was financially successful. But he wasn't interested in amassing money; instead, he collected a sizeable private library.

By far the best thing my father ever did for me was to give me an opportunity, although his idea of an opportunity was a bit different from most people's. He'd once told me about a conversation with his friend, Clyde, who'd made millions in the oil business. His friend complained:

"Ed, I don't know what to do about my kids. Both my boys are away at college, wrecking cars, drinking too much, and generally messing up."

"Well, trouble is they haven't had the opportunities you had," said my dad.

"What are you talking about? I never had *any* opportunities."

"You had the opportunity of coming to Oklahoma on your own at seventeen. You took a job driving a nitroglycerine truck because the pay was high even though it was so dangerous. You had to scratch in rough times. You had the opportunity of becoming a man at an early age. You're denying your sons that opportunity."

During the Depression, of all times, the financial rollercoaster had taken us back up. When the time came, my parents were able to send me to the college of their choice. They chose Carleton College because it was an excellent small co-educational college. But it was understood that the minute my education was completed, I was on my own.

I looked forward to that day eagerly.

After college, my fourth job in as many years was in a tarpaper shack on a construction site in Texas. The job had sounded positively executive over a fancy lunch with the big boss. But in the tarpaper shack I ended up taking dictation from four men.

The nearby small town was full of retired railroad conductors, and that was all. What kind of place was this for a young lady who owned two pairs of alligator shoes, the Gucci loafers of their day?

My father and I had breakfast together in this little town.

"Dad, I can't stand this place."

As the only living daughter of a top executive with a large oil company, I expected something like, "Well, sweetie, come home." But instead, I heard,

"You don't like this little town because you think you're going to be here the rest of your life. But there are trains going out of here both ways every day."

Of course, I knew what to do. I put an ad in the *New York*

Times to find my dream job; the Big Apple was where I wanted to go. It started, "Phi Beta Kappa stranded in tarpaper shack . . . ."

Put in a crazy ad and you'll get a lot of crazy answers.

As it turns out, I didn't get to New York right away. Instead, I took the next train to Tulsa and landed a job with IBM. For seven years I stayed with "Big Blue," occasionally faking it as an "expert." It wasn't easy. Sometimes IBM was taking a long shot when it counted on me to keep its customers educated and happy. But IBM had no choice. Most IBM men were off fighting in World War II.

After six months' training in Endicott, New York, I worked in the Tulsa office for three years. At my first meeting with the manager, he said, "I have 34 Electric Accounting Machine customers; here are your 17."

And as I learned my way around the business, my Tulsa boss spent less and less time in the office, and more and more on the golf course. He'd leave for a week, with nothing more than a wave of his hand.

Actually, it was the chance of a lifetime. The personnel reports were due. I completed them all, including my own, and mailed them in. Naturally, mine was complimentary. The next time the personnel reports were due, my boss was to be gone two weeks. Again, he told me to take charge. This time my personnel report was worded in superlatives.

Soon the company headquarters in New York asked if I could write. Of course I could. And before long I was promoted to Endicott, New York, where I was to write instruction manuals for machines still on the drawing board. I didn't need adjectives or adverbs, but it was necessary to write with clarity. And sometimes I helped design and label new control panels. It was one assignment where I excelled.

But sometimes I was given assignments where I did have to fake it.

There was a terrifying episode in New Haven when, for lack of anyone better, they sent me to Connecticut as "IBM's Special Representative for Blue Cross Accounts." I could make the machines do tricks even IBM hadn't dreamed of, but my knowledge of accounting was that of a fourth grader. Since I was faking it as an expert, I was in constant fear I'd be discovered. I knew I'd really have to wing it. One word of criticism of me to World Headquarters, and I'd have been o-u-t.

What was this Blue Cross controller talking about, zero-balancing? Although perspiring heavily, I did not remove the jacket to my beautifully tailored wool suit, nor did I remove my "expert" expression. Careful not to say one thing that would divulge my ignorance, I finally made it to the safety of the machine room.

I had a guarded chat with the head of the machine room, who spoke my language, then strolled around to see what was going on. But I was still in a quagmire. In desperation, I glanced heavenward. Someone up there must have seen me. Problem: the company was changing its rates. Solution: a flash of inspiration told me I could send all the billing cards through a machine backwards, thereby misreading a letter as an X-punch. This maneuver saved over four hundred hours of an operator's sorting time.

They thought I was a genius. Now I could afford to ask any dumb question, be of real help. I was out of the quagmire.

Soon I was promoted to World Headquarters in New York City. The brier patches became bigger and deeper. But after years of practice, I began to know I could get out of every one. I even had the temerity to enter a contest for a new machine design, along with fifteen hundred engineers.

At the time I was demonstrating, to anyone who stopped to

view it, the Selective Sequence Electronic Calculator that IBM
had on display. One of the first computers, it filled an entire room
on Manhattan's 57th Street with vacuum tubes and relays. Its main
feat at the time was to calculate the distance from the earth to the
moon at any time during the moon's orbit, and it could make this
calculation in a tiny fraction of the time required by any other
method.

My design used components of the SSEC to calculate toll
charges for telephone calls, and then bill them to the customer.
Breathless with anticipation, I heard from my spies that I was tied
for first place. Later I dropped to third. My machine didn't win
because Bell Telephone's Research Lab in New Jersey had a
machine on its drawing board very similar to mine.

First prize had been a diamond watch. Third prize was a short-
wave radio-phonograph. The fact that I could tune in to Nairobi
whenever I wanted didn't make it a more exciting prize. I shipped
it off to Oklahoma as a present for my father who'd become a short
wave radio buff.

During those IBM years, I developed a lot of confidence,
perseverance, and a compulsive determination to succeed once I'd
started something. Thank heaven my father didn't say to me,
"Sweetie, come home." Thank heaven he gave me the opportunity
to build up my own muscle so I'd always be able to get out of brier
patches, especially the giant one in which I found myself in 1970
at the age of 50.

6.

THE
RIGHT PLACE

The subject of nose reconstruction wasn't constantly on my mind at home in Minneapolis. I was too busy. But whenever I'd come to Madison for a checkup, the subject ballooned in my mind and it became my only concern. After all, I had to fulfill the vow I'd made after my two-hour breakdown at the Ivy Inn: that I would come out of the nose surgery looking better than ever.

I continued to scan magazines to see if I could find a model superior to my former nose, and I hungrily read every article I could find on cosmetic surgery. If I was going to have a face lift, an eye job—in fact, the whole works—then I was going to know as much as possible beforehand.

But I didn't want to bother Dr. Mohs about it until the time was ripe, because there were always so many patients waiting to see him.

Finally, by late February, the end of the waiting period was near, and I could hardly wait. Again, I went to Dr. Mohs for a checkup. Those were the days of bouffant hairdos, which were extremely hard to maintain. My operator had already recombed mine twice that week.

I wore a new geranium-red dress, and looked and felt my best as I chatted with others in the waiting room. Then Dr. Mohs called me in.

"I want to compliment you on your reaction in the face of adversity," he said. *Adversity?* Who'd said anything about adversity? When he pared my nose away, he hadn't acted as though disaster had struck. I'd have sworn he thought he was just trimming toenails.

"I've been spending a fortune in the beauty shop."

"Keep it up." He smiled.

Oh, I loved this kind of advice. But at last I felt the time was ripe.

"Who is the best plastic surgeon in the world?"

I hoped it was someone in an exotic locale. "Vienna" repeated itself in my head. I could see myself sipping wine at a sidewalk cafe during my lazy convalescence, a mysterious figure swathed in a mauve chiffon scarf.

His reply was rather matter-of-fact. "Because I do so much skin cancer removal, a team of plastic surgeons right here in Madison probably have repaired more noses—defective in the same way that yours is defective—than anyone in the world. Talk to Dr. Gordon Davenport." As soon as I got home I phoned to make an appointment with Dr. Davenport. So much for Vienna.

I'd never found a magazine nose as nice as my own, and I knew Dr. Davenport would need a model to go by. I rummaged through attic drawers and dug out some old pictures of myself. The photographer's lighting had made me look glamorous, especially with my best feature intact.

With my photo collection in a manila folder, I flew from Minneapolis to Madison to get his proposal for nose reconstruction and wrinkle removal. Since it was only a consultation, I went alone.

Dr. Davenport's waiting room resembled those of other doctors in private practice, only in better taste, carpeted, with comfortable sofas and chairs.It was an early spring day, but winter hadn't given up its fight yet in Wisconsin. The doctor's lamps were softly lit, their warm glow illuminating the lovely prints on the walls. I felt upper class just to be sitting there, and euphoric about getting to a place where they could make me beautiful. If someone was going to build something in the middle of my face, I was glad to see that he had a sense of artistry.

Soon a nurse led me into his office.

He shook my hand and smiled. "How do you do, Mrs. Shuck? Dr. Mohs has told me about you." He introduced me to a young resident.

"Now, let's see what we have here."

Dr. Davenport painstakingly went over the nose defects and my forehead skin with a tiny metal ruler, marked off in what I supposed were millimeters.

The young resident gently pinched my cheek.

"Mrs. Shuck's skin's been irradiated by X-rays," Dr. Davenport said. "Her cheek skin can't be used; it's 'floppy tissue.' Too, the wounds made by Mohs look smaller than they actually are."

He was very deliberate, completely unhurried, and so intent on what he was doing that I kept the photos in their manila folder. I didn't want to interrupt his concentration. I'd show them to him later.

He turned back to his examination and spent a long time looking at the skin on my forehead, measuring and marking off a piece of it on the left side.

"Yes," he said, "I recommend a forehead flap."

"A *what*?"

"I'd get a piece of skin from the left side of your forehead to grow onto the remaining portion of your nose. It'll cover the larger and smaller holes, and also the part of the tip that's missing.

"Now, Mrs. Shuck, it is a rather involved operation, because the forehead skin cannot simply be severed from your forehead and sewn to your nose. It could die if we did that." He continued matter-of-factly, seemingly unaware of my growing panic.

"So the forehead skin will be severed from your forehead on only three sides. The top side will stay attached to a strip of skin lifted from your shaved scalp. The other end of the strip of skin will stay attached to your scalp just above your opposite ear.

"Until the forehead skin can establish circulation with your nose, it will be kept alive by a blood supply coming from this strip of shaved scalp. This scalp strip will carry a blood supply to the forehead skin for the three weeks it takes it to grow onto your nose. When it does, we'll sever it and put the scalp strip back where it came from."

"Oh, no. My hair is my best remaining feature."

"We won't shave your entire head, just four inches back from your hairline, and only from behind the forehead piece to just above the opposite ear. In other words we'll give you a temporary receding hairline."

"But won't there be a bare strip of skull when you lift the shaved skin?"

"We'll cover it with a thin piece of skin taken from your thigh. Since the nose needs a lining, the forehead skin will be lined in a preliminary operation, also with a thin piece of skin from your leg."

"I don't really understand, but I'm not sure I want you to repeat that."

Good God, how sickening! I just hoped I wouldn't throw up.

"Here. I'll show you a picture." He got out a surgery textbook and showed me an illustration.

From the schematic drawing, I could see that the sides of the patient's forehead skin were stitched down the sides of the nose, the bottom stitched around the tip. The top of the forehead skin was still attached to the end of the shaved scalp strip at what had been the hairline. The other end of the scalp strip was still attached to the scalp just above the right ear. Apparently, the scalp strip had been tied into a tube, narrower in the middle, so that the patient could peek around it as it swung from above the right ear to the bridge of the nose.

"Are you sure my hair will grow back?"

"Yes. In fact, it'll start sprouting from the scalp strip while you're still in the hospital. After the surgeries, you can wear a wig until your hair grows out."

"How will you get me back together? The scalp strip back on my head?"

"In about three weeks, we'll cut half way through the scalp strip, at the point where it's attached to the forehead skin. In about another week we'll cut the rest of the way through the scalp strip. We take the scalp strip away from the nose skin in these two stages so that circulation from the scalp won't be removed suddenly."

He shrugged. "Then it's just a matter of putting the scalp strip back where it came from. In this last operation we also attached the top edge of the forehead skin to the nose, up on the bridge."

With a shaved head and that hair-sprouting scalp strip dangling across my face, I'll be more frightening than Dracula. How will DeWitt bear to look at me? If I die on the operating table, is this the way he'll remember me? Dracula, the mother of his three children?

"Since you're from out of town, you'll stay in the hospital six weeks. It's a five-surgery procedure. For three of the operations, we'll give you general anesthesia."

When I was a child, doctors said I shouldn't have general anesthetics because I had a leaky heart valve. Later exams had shown my heart normal, but at the moment this old message about anesthesia was playing back loud and clear.

"Isn't all that anesthesia dangerous?"

"No. We sometimes put burn victims under four times in a week."

"Is this surgery terribly painful?"

"Some patients have felt some discomfort, but none have complained of much pain."

That was hard to believe.

"You'll come back for two trimmings this year."

I didn't even want to know what he meant by "trimmings." I couldn't absorb any more. I felt weak. Perspiration was rolling down my body. My Arrid X-tra Dry had quit working.

"Would you like to look at some pictures of my former nose?"

"No. They wouldn't help. You'll have an acceptable nose, but it can't be like your old one."

"Acceptable?"

"Well, from time to time, someone sitting next to you may think, 'There's something peculiar about that woman's nose.'"

To think I'd imagined that a nose repair would be so simple they could do a face lift at the same time.

I wobbled out to the appointment desk on jello-like legs, and set the appointment for April 19, 1971, to start the forehead flap surgeries. It would be six weeks away, but it was impossible to accommodate the precise scheduling of the five surgeries any earlier.

I hurried out to make the afternoon plane back to Minneapolis. A taxi sped me to the airport, the photos in the manila folder clutched in my damp hand.

I missed the 3:10 plane by seconds; it was five hours till the next one. My book would normally have been a page-turner, but I couldn't concentrate and finally put it down. I couldn't think of anything other than a stubble-covered tube of living skin. And in the public airport lobby there wasn't a private spot where I could permit myself even a half-hour nervous breakdown.

Who in the world had devised such an obscene surgical procedure? And how had the first patient looked afterward? Had someone actually volunteered for such a thing?

Five-thirty finally came and I went into the airport dining room. I saw an unfamiliar woman sitting at a table and asked if I could sit with her. Everything had been piling up inside me since I left Dr. Davenport. I had to talk to someone—anyone.

I ordered a martini.

In a long, torrential outpouring mixed with tears, I told her what had happened to my nose, and about how frightened I'd been by Dr. Davenport's proposal.

She made no comment.

Unfazed by her coolness, I still needed to get out all that was troubling me. "I have another problem. My aunt died recently, and left me some money. Since I didn't know her very well, maybe I should give it to her brother. He's been closer to her but I do know my medical trips are going to be expensive. What do you think?"

"Do you really *need* the money?"

"No."

I really should be less interested in myself. "By the way, where do you live?"

"Colony Springs. I'm the wife of the minister for Calvary Baptist Church."

And there I sat with my martini.

On the plane, I mentally designed a contraption to conceal me from view during the six-week forehead flap ordeal.

I'd use an umbrella to carry over my head; to its outer edge I'd sew a ten-inch-wide strip of chiffon, long enough to completely encircle the umbrella. Maybe a nice Japanese parasol. Its spokes are only about two inches apart on the rim when it's opened and I could easily sew the wide chiffon strip to those spokes.

When I opened the umbrella, the chiffon strip would drop down and hide me. And I'd use two layers of chiffon for the drop: white on the outside, and black on the inside.

My fantasy continued: I know this'll work. People can visit with me, but I'll be hidden from them. They'll only see white chiffon. I'll be able to see all the bald heads on the outside, but they can't possibly see mine.

Now my thoughts became less fantastic: And I'm definitely going to accept the money from my aunt's estate. I'll use it to phone friends all over the country during my hospital stay. And if things get desperate, I'll send for Peg, my wonderful, long-time friend.

These plans made me feel far less helpless. I'd have some control over my life during the surgeries. I could make those six weeks in the hospital almost pleasant.

That evening I landed in the bosom of my entire family: John and Ted were home on spring break. I told them right away about my planned umbrella device. Almost everyone looked puzzled.

But Ted, with his engineering mind, understood exactly what I'd designed. He said, "Sure, that'll work just great."

Of course it would. After absorbing the first awful shock of the forehead flap procedure while stranded in the airport lobby, I grew sure everything would work just great.

7.

DETOUR

DeWitt suggested I get a second opinion from our regular clinic after he heard my description of the forehead flap. For many years we'd gone to a well-known clinic for annual checkups. We'd go with friends and make a party of it.

Each patient there is assigned a consulting internist who does the general examination. He recommends specialists to be seen and tests to be given, then later ties the results together in a summation interview. As part of my yearly exam, my internist always sent me to the dermatology department where a doctor checked my skin. My present story had begun ten months before in May of 1970, when I'd complained to a dermatologist during my yearly exam that my nose had been crusting and bleeding. He had merely cauterized it. Now, the following March, I phoned Dr. Morgan, my internist at the clinic.

"Good morning, Mrs. Shuck, how are you?"

"Not too well. Last May your dermatology department missed large skin cancers on my forehead and chin and also on my nose. A few months later they were removed by Dr. Fred Mohs. He's at

University Hospital and Clinic in Madison, Wisconsin. Now my nose needs reconstruction."

Since I'd heard that DeWitt's company sends more employees to this clinic for yearly exams than any other, and I was sure Dr. Morgan recognized my name, I hoped to get red carpet treatment. My next sentence was more conciliatory.

"Since then I've seen Dr. Gordon Davenport, a plastic surgeon in Madison. He's recommended a forehead flap, scheduled for April. But, first, I'd like to find out what your plastic surgeons think."

"If you can come tomorrow, I'll arrange an appointment with Dr. Henry Lang. He's our head of plastic surgery."

"I can be there by eleven."

"Fine. Come around to my office first. I'd like to see you."

The next morning I walked into the main clinic building. It always reminded me of a luxurious office building from New York's Rockefeller Center that had been air lifted to the Midwest. Contemporary sculpture enhanced the building's exterior and interior walls. The halls and waiting rooms were huge with enormously high ceilings that made them seem even larger. Uniformed elevator operators stood at sharp attention and were meticulously groomed, always courteous.

The tremendous waiting rooms were usually filled to capacity. I supposed a thousand patients must be going through the clinic at any one time, everything running with clock-like efficiency.

After being greeted by Dr. Morgan, I was quickly shown into Dr. Lang's office, which looked remarkably like all the other clinic offices I'd seen, with chairs and desks of the best quality and such medical equipment as necessary. Everything looked new and beautifully maintained. In all my visits, I never saw anything in a doctor's office that would identify it as belonging to a specific doctor: no personal books, pictures, rugs, or plants. Perhaps this gave the use of office space more flexibility?

No doctor or medical group likes to admit overlooking a serious problem and I'm sure Dr. Lang had been alerted to the dermatology department's mistake. New in his post as head of plastic surgery, he probably saw me as the perfect patient on whom he could practice being a hero.

He took one look. "No. A four-stage forehead flap is using too big a gun. I can get the same result with a simple one-step operation, using a piece of your cheek."

"But Dr. Davenport said my cheek can't be used. He called it 'floppy tissue' because my skin's been x-rayed for acne."

"Nonsense. I think I'll probably use the inside of your upper lip for a nose lining, tunneling it up."

"Dr. Davenport did say my new nose couldn't be perfect, certainly not like my old nose. But that it would be acceptable."

"I don't think you'll have a funny looking nose."

What a handsome, assured man! Assured possibly to the point of arrogance but I can forgive a little arrogance. Maybe it's just evidence that he knows his stuff.

Tennis players like to watch tennis matches. Golfers enjoy golf tournaments. And salesmen like to hear a good sales pitch. That's probably why the old saying is true: salesmen are the most easily sold people in the world.

Maybe my years of selling IBM machines put me at a disadvantage. Sometimes, feeling nostalgic, I'd invite the Fuller Brush Man in, just to hear a good sales pitch.

I heard one that day. Dr. Lang said exactly what I wanted to hear.

I was uneasy, though, about Dr. Davenport's having described my cheek skin as unsuitable for reconstruction. I decided to go talk to Dr. Morgan about such a difference of opinion on such an essential point.

"Dr. Davenport—the plastic surgeon in Madison who proposed the forehead flap—said my cheek skin can't be used because it's been irradiated; that it's 'floppy tissue.' Do you think Dr. Lang could be using a compromise method?"

"No, Dr. Lang would never do such a thing."

I breathed a sigh of relief. After all, Dr. Morgan had also been used by a President of the United States.

I made an appointment at the clinic for the simple surgery, and canceled my appointment for the forehead flap.

That evening I talked over my day with DeWitt.

"Well, Dr. Lang told me that he could repair my nose in one simple operation, using a piece of my cheek."

"Didn't Dr. Davenport think cheek skin was a bad idea?"

"I know, but I talked it over with Dr. Morgan and he assured me Dr. Lang wouldn't use a compromise method."

"And Dr. Lang wants to use the inside of your upper lip to line your nose?"

"That's what he said. It's a novel idea, maybe something recently devised."

"Well, the clinic does seem to be on the cutting edge of medical care." He laughed and put his arm around me. "No pun intended."

I was unsettled, my stomach queasy, during our drive to the clinic for the upcoming simple surgery. Surely they weren't butchers at this famous clinic. I hoped this was just routine cold feet that I'd have prior to any surgery, or did my subconscious know something?

In my hospital room that evening, I remembered my sister, Marjorie, dying after a tonsillectomy, a simple operation even back then. I remembered the childhood warning against my undergoing anesthesia.

I looked out my window at a neon sign that read, "DAHLQUIST."

If only I'll be here to read that sign again tomorrow evening.

I said the Twenty-third Psalm. It was the most affirmative, heartening prayer I knew: "The Lord is my Shepherd, I shall not want . . . ."

In the morning, I was wheeled up to the operating room. My shaking, sweaty hands gripped the sides of the gurney. After an injection, I seemed to disappear.

When I awoke, I was astonished.

There was the DAHLQUIST sign. Relief swept over me. If that sign's still there, I must still be here too.

I'd always been an admitted coward, insisting on novocaine for the tiniest dental filling. After John was born, I went to see my doctor and demanded he make it his personal mission in life to devise a less torturous way of producing children, pounding my fist on his desk so hard I bruised it.

Plastic surgery, by contrast, seemingly was painless. I just had a nice nap during the surgery and didn't even have to help my "caregivers."

In my clinic room that night DeWitt and I watched the greatest prize fight of the year on television. I winced as boxers exchanged blows, but otherwise I was comfortable, completely relaxed. Nothing hurt.

Dr. Lang stopped by. "Everything went well. I worked very hard for four-and-a-half hours. I'll need to do just a little more work on the very tip in about three months, probably under a local."

I took a look at myself in the bathroom mirror. Stitches closed the "smile" line on my right cheek, and ran back and forth across my nose. I looked as though one of those boxers had socked me on the lower right side of my face and upper lip. Still, I wasn't in any pain.

At about nine that evening I was given a sleeping pill and got very drowsy. Relaxed, overjoyed to have the surgery behind me, I could have slept comfortably in just about any position, even on my back or left side. But, as in any hospital, my door was left wide open, dim hall lights streamed in, and nurses talked in normal voices at the nearby nursing station. Periodically one would come into the room to check my IV, blood pressure, and pulse, so I was able to sleep only fitfully.

A day or two later I asked for an aspirin, more to relieve the general boredom than to ease my slight headache. A tiny nurse came in with a huge, shiny steel hypodermic syringe.

"This is what has been prescribed for pain."

"Oh, no, you don't. I don't want that."

She all but attacked me with it; only my winning a tug-of-war with the bed sheets saved me.

It was hard to eat with the lining of my upper lip gone, yet I was served a normal tray with solid food.

Over the phone, a friend said, "Get a turkey baster. You can use it to suck up liquids or mashed potatoes and squirt them to the back of your mouth."

So I requested a turkey baster. Repeatedly. To no avail.

"I believe I'll call Marian Stauffer, the wife of Dr. Stauffer here at the clinic," I finally told a nurse. "I'm sure she'll bring me her turkey baster."

Magically, a turkey baster was delivered to my room within minutes.

I looked a little better each day. After a week, stitches were removed. I was given penicillin for possible infection, and we returned home. The swelling and discoloration were almost gone. I continued taking penicillin.

Three days later I became feverish, then so chilled I couldn't get warm. I broke out in purple hives. I called our family doctor. His colleague instructed me to come to his office. DeWitt drove me there and sat in the waiting room while I saw the doctor. I was weak, hardly able to make it in to see him.

"You go to a fancy clinic and then you come to us to bail you out," he said. "Now here's a prescription for prednisone. You're to take it for thirty days in gradually lessening dosages. You'll finish by taking only a quarter of a tablet for three days. The dosages for each of the thirty days are to be taken in strict accordance with the schedule I've marked out on this instruction sheet. Don't stop taking it suddenly or you could die. Understand?"

I was too limp to respond, barely alert enough to comprehend what he was saying. He helped me to the waiting room, and stopped when he saw DeWitt stand up.

He turned to me, "I do feel terribly sorry for you, Mrs. Shuck."

Our children were still on their spring school break, so we decided to take a family vacation to La Jolla, California. We stayed at a beach and tennis club. Vacationers are seldom in their rooms, so the rooms were Spartan, dreary.

The vacation began dismally. For several days, the penicillin reaction confined me to bed. I hadn't brought my Micropore tape, so reading was out, and there was no TV.

John and DeWitt went to play golf at La Costa, an elegant spa up the way. "What was it like?"

"Very new-rich," said DeWitt, "You wouldn't like it at all."

"Wanna bet? I'd love to try it."

In a few days, I did manage to stagger into an elegant ladies' apparel shop to try on every garment. I've wondered since why they let me try them on; I was still covered with purple penicillin hives. Maybe they hated to hurt a smallpox victim's feelings? Or maybe they fumigated the place a little later in the day.

Soon I had my hair done and things got better fast. We had drinks in the wonderful Marine Room, the ocean waves pounding against the windows. A fire was roaring in the fireplace. I have great respect for alcohol's unsheathed blade, but there is something comforting about enjoying it in moderation. Words flow, ideas are expressed that otherwise go unexpressed. People are closer. That evening was one I will always cherish.

Dr. Lang's surgery had closed the smaller hole on the left side of my nose. But the right side, as well as the tip, needed more work. His novel idea also left the inside of my upper lip stiff. My mouth had lost some of its agility. I didn't mention it, because my family would have died laughing. I could talk just as fast and say as much as before—and certainly I did—but it was hard to pronounce certain words distinctly.

It was also difficult to open my mouth wide enough to eat something thick. "I'm afraid my hamburger and BLT days are over," I told Ellen.

Three months later, in June, I went back for my nose touch-up at the clinic. Ted drove me there; DeWitt was to join me later. Since this clinic is a teaching institution, a group of interns often accompany a doctor. That morning Dr. Lang had his troops arrayed behind him.

He looked at my nose. "Whew," he said, then paused, as he tapped on his metal clipboard, "I think, if you stick with us, we can still give you a nose."

If I stick with them, what did that mean?

"I'll bring some skin from the middle of your forehead down

under the skin between your eyes and onto the bridge of your nose," Dr. Lang said.

"Wait a minute: what do you mean, *if* I stick with you? If I must, I can come back sixteen times. Do you *really* think you can give me a nose?"

"Yes, I'm determined."

My instincts were screaming that something was wrong here, but bewilderment and blind trust had completely overcome good judgment. Instead of leaving, I made the appointment for surgery the next morning.

The worst part of any operation is the anticipation. For the first surgery, I'd been lucky enough to be taken right up to the operating room at eight in the morning; paralyzed with shots, I was unable to consider fleeing.

This time, because of the surgery schedule, I had to stay in my room until eleven in the morning. DeWitt waited with me, and together we worked a crossword puzzle. I'd found I could concentrate on such puzzles even when I couldn't read with comprehension.

Finally an attendant came for me and off I went.

As I went under the anesthetic, I had a dream of DeWitt and Dr. Lang lifting arms and palms upward as they shrugged their shoulders, as if to say, "Well, it'll never work."

A dirge-like tune in a minor key accompanied their gesture. "Tuum tuum ti tum . . . Tuum ti tum . . . Tuum tumm ti tum . . . Tuuuuuuuuuuuuuum. . . ."

Each Tuum tumm ti tumm was lower on the scale.

Was my subconscious still trying to tell me something?

The operation was another lengthy one: three-and-a-half hours.

This time, I came out of the anesthetic while still in the operating room, and I distinctly heard Dr. Lang talking to the surgical team.

"I doubt very much that this will do it."

I was sure this remark was no dream, but something I'd heard while fully conscious.

I later discovered that during this operation, Dr. Lang had cut a vertical strip of skin about a half-inch wide from the middle of my forehead, tunneled it under skin between my eyes, and sewed it to the bridge of my nose. However, the forehead skin didn't reach far enough to cover the tip.

Why in the world didn't he MEASURE the forehead strip before doing the surgery? No wonder I'd overheard that remark.

Stitches ran down the middle of my forehead and around the forehead skin now on my nose. The skin between my eyes was stretched, distorted, swollen.

For eight days, I shared a room with a girl from Montana who'd had a melanoma removed from her scalp. I felt exceedingly sorry for her. She cried a lot, and ate almost nothing. Grafting skin back onto her scalp was painful, and I suffered with her as they dressed the grafts.

But, again, I had no pain. I couldn't tape my glasses to my forehead to read, so I was bored. I taped my roommate's get-well cards onto the wall by her bed.

"How can you be so nonchalant about being deformed?" she asked.

Without thinking, I whirled around to face her. "Because I've been through much worse." I was astounded I'd said it.

I was referring to Marjorie's death, a childhood tragedy whose effect that had long outlived the actual event, but one that had also made the world seem forever after a delightful place where nothing really too bad could ever happen again. And for that instant I was thankful that an early experience with tragedy had trained me to take some momentary pain in stride.

On my sixth day in the hospital, John and Ted drove to the clinic and we had a great visit on a small balcony. They'd smuggled me a little bottle of bourbon. We talked about John's plans to spend the summer going up the Nile with a friend. Native style. They also planned to come back through Europe. All this on a tight budget.

"Aren't you worried you'll get yourself caught in the middle of an Arab-Israeli war?"

"No, my Jewish friends tell me I'm so blond that neither side will mistake me for the enemy and shoot me."

We laughed.

Ted was about to leave for Gold Lake Camp in Colorado, where he'd been a long-time counselor. "I've got a new bow and arrow set," he said, "it's eight feet long. I'll be able to start a new class in marksmanship."

"How are you going to get it to Colorado?"

"You know Ted," John said, "he'll arrive at the airline counter with more equipment than the Camp has. The airline people will say he can't take it on the plane, but Ted'll stand there, all helpless, as if to say 'I'm your problem.' They'll give up and send his gear around to special handling. It'll arrive in Colorado on the same plane with him."

After eight days my eyes were still discolored and swollen. Not a pretty sight. Before I left, Dr. Lang took out the stitches and applied an antibiotic cream. He told me I could put on makeup in a few days. I was to come back in August for another touch-up.

Four or five days after my return home, we were invited to a large, fancy dinner dance. I couldn't *wait* to get to that party.

I called my hostess, a good friend, to make little noises about how terrible I looked. "Really, Marge, I do look awful."

"Well, we'd love to have you but I want you to be comfortable," she said. "What do you really want to do?"

"Oh, I'd just love to come, if you think it's okay."

"Of course. I was hoping you'd say that."

I carefully applied liquid makeup. With the stitches out, the scar on my forehead had become a fine line, almost unnoticeable with the makeup, but my eyes were still discolored and swollen. I looked like the victim of a mugging, but I put a larger flesh-colored bandage on my nose and went to the party.

Somehow it didn't bother me to appear in public. There were few mirrors, lots of other people to engage my attention, and I was always on the inside looking out. In any case, I knew it was only a temporary disfigurement.

I had a great time at the dance. My host was witty and a fabulous dancer. Probably having no other option, his wife had seated me on his right. I wore a beautiful new gown, just my shade of blue. Contrary to the usual arrangement, the zipper on the skirt hooked at the waist, then zipped down to the hem.

Suddenly, during the execution of an ambitious, dervish-like whirl, my skirt unzipped, hem-to-waist, exposing my girdle.

I grabbed at the zipper and yanked it down. For a moment I thought no one had noticed, but my partner was in hysterics. This little accident was far more embarrassing than running about with a nose that was under construction.

Once I was back with family and good friends, I blocked the plastic surgeries out of my mind. For every week I had spent at plastic surgery, I spent three months in the normal world doing my usual thing.

On Fridays I met my gossiping bridge foursome; on Tuesdays I worked at the women's clinic and attended a board meeting. I had lunch with the sewing club that didn't sew, and we went out a lot socially.

My eyes weren't discolored for long after the second surgery.

But the skin between my eyes was thickened and stretched out of place. I looked as if I were frowning, perplexed. This change in expression bothered me far more than my tape-covered nose. I assumed Dr. Lang would correct the distortion. After all, I was in the hands of the head of plastic surgery at a world-renowned clinic.

In August, I went back for more reconstruction. There was still no tip.

The large notch in the right side of my nose was ugly.

The day before surgery, Dr. Lang had suggested a local anesthetic and mulled over two possibilities for getting more skin onto my nose.

"I might just use skin from a finger. It would be tied up to your nose until the finger skin establishes circulation and attaches itself."

He sighed, shook his head, flipped through a book.

"Then again, I just might use skin from your left cheek instead. You see, I've been reading . . . ."

The knot in my stomach twisted a little tighter. Did he plan to bring that text into surgery with him?

About half an hour before the surgery a young man came into my hospital room to give me a shot of demerol in the arm. I knew what little effect demerol had on me during childbirth.

"Give me another shot in my other arm."

"Oh, that might not make you feel so good," he said.

"I've got two arms; why not use both of them? I know it'll make me feel a lot better."

He gave me a shot in the other arm.

I was wheeled up to a fascinating experience, right into the movie *M*A*S*H*. Better, because I wasn't a spectator. I had the starring role. The scene opened in a hallway, where I was allowed to rest for a good half hour.

Please, dear God, don't let my shots wear off. The Lord is . . . The Lord is my . . . What's wrong? I can't seem to juggle the words of the Twenty-third Psalm into their correct sequence.

A fellow patient was prone on his cart. Tubes ran out from under sheets and into jars. I looked away, said a prayer for him too.

Men in white coats argued. "Well, we don't know where his chart is. Dermatology had it last. It's up to them to find his chart."

I hoped the patient was asleep.

In spite of the Demerol, I was wide awake, very aware as they wheeled me into surgery.

They scrubbed my finger and my face with an antibacterial soap. Dr. Lang sat on a stool in the corner, watching everything, and stroking his chin.

"Go ahead. Scrub my thumb." I said.

"Inseparable my nose and thumb" became a joke original with me. Over and over I repeated it to the operating theater. I'd never been more clever.

At the last moment, Dr. Lang decided to use a strip of skin from my unused cheek. Out of it he would make a flap lined with some skin from my leg. One end would stay attached to my cheek, the other could grow onto the tip of my nose. In a week or two he'd detach the flap from my cheek. He'd shape the tip from the cheek skin growing there.

He cut into my cheek, forgetting to inject the deadener.

"Novocaine," I said, "remember?"

He'd told me before that local anesthetic couldn't be used in the nose itself because it makes the tissues puff up and become distorted so that he couldn't accurately judge what he was doing. But I knew he could put it in the cheek.

When he tried to decide which leg to use for a flap lining, I said, "The one with the thicker skin, the left leg, of course." I was glad I hadn't added, "You dunce."

The Demerol made the experience unreal; any pain was far away. The movie starring me was turning out to be a spectacular show.

By this time, I imagined myself an unsurpassed comedian. "Promise not to touch my heels; I'm not through kicking them up."

Dr. Lang would call out "hook," then "scalpel," then "catgut," then "nylon."

"I don't have any nylon for suture," a nurse said.

"I don't have any nylon for suture." Dr. Lang mimicked her perfectly in a feminine voice.

Ready to take the split thickness graft from my leg, they discovered the instrument that removes the skin in a net-like layer had been misplaced.

"Well, hand me that razor blade," Dr. Lang said.

He used it. Expertly.

After two hours, he'd finished; I was wheeled downstairs.

The surgery had hurt a little, but it was as if it had hurt someone else. I hadn't cared about anything; they could have sawed off my head without a word of protest from me. And there wasn't the awful pre-surgery fear that I might not wake up to see the DAHLQUIST sign.

I decided local anesthetics were the way to go.

The next day I went home to wait for the cheek flap to attach itself. A large piece of white gauze was taped over my nose, and the adjacent left cheek. Dr. Lang still hadn't fixed the misshapen skin between my eyes that made me look dismayed. And with the removal of skin from my left cheek, my face looked skeletal.

Fixing up a nose was clearly like redecorating a room. It had to look worse before it could look better.

But now, at any rate, I was back once again in the pleasant outside world, where the memory of surgery quickly melted away. I did shopping, had out-of-town friends to dinner, and was involved in daily living.

After eight days I went back to the clinic, where technicians determined that the circulation between my cheek skin and nose was established.

"I can form the tip tomorrow morning," Dr. Lang said. "Then I'll be through. Your nose will be complete. It'll just amount to peanuts."

"Really?"

"Sure. I can do it under a local anesthetic. You won't even have to be hospitalized."

"How long will it take?"

"Only twenty minutes."

Ecstatic, I checked into the top hotel's best room, ordered up a screwdriver, poured it over ice, and sat down to watch TV. I munched away on a can of cashews, my favorites.

I was going first class. And how I loved those local anesthetics. Another crazy movie with me in it, and then I'd have graduated. I'd reached the end of a long tunnel.

I toasted myself with my screwdriver. "To paradise."

I called DeWitt to tell him the news.

"That's great, sweetie. I'll drive over early tomorrow morning. I'll be waiting in the hospital lobby when your surgery's over."

The next morning, I checked into the hospital. Directed to the surgical floor, I was handed a hospital gown and paper slippers. I sat on a stool and began to undress. "The hospital's filled," someone in the next dressing room said, "there aren't any more rooms."

Was lack of hospital space the reason I was entering surgery on foot and wide awake this time? Eight days ago I was on a gurney and all shot up with Demerol. I shrugged and kicked off my shoes. After all, it was only a twenty-minute procedure this time.

Dr. Lang "hooked," "scalpeled," "catgutted," and "nyloned," for what seemed an eternity. I watched the clock on the wall. The minute hand circled time after time in slow motion. One hundred and twenty times.

This time I wasn't doing any clever ad-libbing. This time I was on a bad trip with no drugs.

There's that line in the Twenty-third Psalm, "Thou preparest a table before me in the presence of mine enemies." Surely David hadn't meant an operating table.

Once, between implement changes, I carefully cleared my throat, "I'm going through this for only two reasons," I said through clenched teeth. "One, I can't get down off this table. Two, I'd like a nose."

"Those are two good reasons," quoth Dr. Lang blandly.

Finally, the terrible procedure was over.

I made it down off the table. Scrambled into my clothes as if the building were on fire. Raced for the elevator.

DeWitt would be waiting in the lobby.

A surgical nurse followed me to the elevator. "Didn't you have any sedative?"

"None."

"Next time you insist on it. You could have gone into shock."

Shock? I was too damned angry at Dr. Lang for putting me through such torture to have ever gone into shock.

Just peanuts, indeed.

In November, Dr. Lang operated for the fourth time. When I went for stitch removal after this last surgery, he gave me a hand mirror.

"What do you think of your nose? Now, be honest."

"There's still that large notch and no tip."

"Yes, that's our problem."

"No. That's *my* problem. And what are you going to do about it?"

I was to come back in January.

Only two weeks after the last surgery, we were invited to spend Thanksgiving as houseguests of dear friends in Keokuk, our former hometown.

I felt that my face looked cadaverous, all carved up. The skin between my eyes was still distorted. I wore Micropore tape on my nose to cover the defects, but it couldn't hide the other scars. Even so, back in the company of long-standing friends, I felt safe, loved, cared-for.

Back in Minneapolis, I was frantically, furiously busy getting ready for Christmas. Just decorating our large home was a three-day job. There were cards to be chosen, notes to be written; gift shopping, package wrapping and mailing: extra holiday cooking and baking; and readying the guest rooms. John and Ted would be home, and DeWitt's sister and her husband were coming from Kansas City.

For the first time since Dr. Lang started, I had a leaden, sinking feeling. It was almost constant. I'd been sailing along; now I was dragging anchor. I knew these things took time, but more and more I was becoming convinced that things weren't working out after all. Maybe they never would.

One day I went down to the basement wrapping table to do up some packages and crumpled into a chair. Alone, I sobbed, and wept bitter, salty tears.

Was I always going to be ugly? Always?

"Can you come up here, Mrs. Shuck?" someone called down.

Suddenly, I was so exhausted I couldn't answer. But in a few minutes, I bathed my eyes in the cool water of the laundry sink and managed to pull myself up the basement stairs to the kitchen.

At a holiday dinner party, a friend asked who was doing my surgery.

"A specialist at the clinic where we go," I said. "Sometimes I wonder if he knows what he's doing."

"I can imagine how you feel. You've been at this a long time."

"He's head of plastic surgery there, but sometimes people get to high places more on the strength of ambition than talent. Sometimes I think this could be true of Dr. Lang. He's so proud, so arrogant, so aggressively positive."

"It's strange that you should say that. We know him socially. It's exactly what my husband thinks. He can't stand him."

The holiday season was so busy that I couldn't spare many daylight hours worrying, but my nights became a dark sea of anxiety. I clung to the Twenty-third Psalm like a life preserver.

One sleepless night, I did some calculations.

Four hundred dollars' worth of Micropore tape, retail, will last me the rest of my life if I live to be eighty. Maybe if I buy a share or two of Minnesota Mining stock, I can get it wholesale. Then I can live a lot longer.

The tape was a lifesaver, and I hoped they never stopped making it.

It was comforting to have a good friend near the clinic.

"I have a friend whose husband's a neurosurgeon at the clinic," she said over the phone. "She had her nose rebuilt there. Her plastic surgeon was Dr. Gaston, who's been there for years."

"How many surgeries did she have, do you know?"

"Three. I know she got discouraged and was depressed for months but now her nose is better looking than it was in the first place."

Why hadn't Dr. Lang done her surgery? After all, he was the

department head, even though Dr. Gaston had more seniority. Maybe the senior plastic surgeon was a personal friend. But what a relief to hear this patient's newly-restored nose was even better looking than her old one.

I went to see Dr. Lang again in January. It was now 1972, and I looked just as I had in November 1971.

Dr. Lang had an older plastic surgeon with him. When he introduced him as Dr. Gaston, my spirits began to rise.

Dr. Lang sat facing me. Dr. Gaston stood behind him.

"Since I can't do a thing to line Mrs. Shuck's nose satisfactorily," Dr. Lang said, "I can't do another thing."

"Why don't you line a forehead flap," I said, "then build the nose with the lined skin?"

Dr. Gaston smiled broadly at me, and vigorously nodded his head.

Dr. Lang couldn't see the gesture. But I got the message. The senior plastic surgeon felt Dr. Davenport's way was the way to go; that a forehead flap would do it.

"I want you to look at some prostheses," Dr. Lang said.

A plastic nose?

"You've got to be kidding. If they're so great, why didn't you show them to me last March before doing four surgeries? Forget it. I'm perfectly happy with Micropore tape."

"I will not have a patient leave my department wearing tape on her nose."

"Look, just fix the area between my eyes, where you tunneled skin, and take out that bad scar. Try to make my face look the way it used to. That bothers me a lot more than a piece of flesh-colored tape on my nose."

But he resisted and I reluctantly agreed to meet him after lunch in the clinic's prosthesis department.

I'd become frightened; things were not working out, but the plastic nose was beyond frightening. The proposal left me stunned. I felt as though a steel trap were being lowered over me. I had to escape. I all but ran from Dr. Lang's office. I rushed for the nearest phone booth, dropped in a dime, and phoned Dr. Mohs.

"Now they're proposing a plastic nose."

"You'd better come back over here. I'll make an appointment for you tomorrow with Dr. Davenport."

In the phone booth I remembered that four months before, while checking my face for cancers, Dr. Mohs had told me that some plastic surgeons were artists, some were butchers. Why in blue blazes hadn't I pursued that observation further? At least, now, I've escaped the finality of a plastic nose.

I took a relaxed, deep breath,—the first deep breath I'd taken since Dr. Lang made his announcement that he was through.

I also phoned DeWitt. "Dr. Lang tells me he can't do anything more. He's recommending a plastic nose."

"That's terrible. I'll leave right away and meet you in Dr. Lang's office this afternoon. I want to know what's going on."

I nonchalantly strolled off to the hotel dining room to keep a date with my local friend. Greatly relieved after talking with Dr. Mohs, I dawdled over an extra martini and a leisurely lunch. It was the first time in my life that I'd ever kept a doctor waiting; I was a half hour late when I met Dr. Lang to look at the plastic noses.

My reaction is best described in the letter I wrote two days later to Ted and John, both at college:

> My dear boys,
> I just have to tell you the latest. On Monday, I packed my bag and departed for the clinic, equipped to stay for surgery.

Dr. Lang saw me, looked at my nose, and shook his head. He called in another plastic surgeon there and said he could not do one damned thing. I said,

"All right. I've been anticipating this. Just clear up the area between my eyes where you tunneled the forehead skin and take out that bad scar." In other words, I wanted him to clean up his mess. (Sound familiar, boys?)

I did go downstairs with him to see a Dr. Ramirez, the man who concocts these things. I passed the assortment of noses, the collection of ears, the array of thumbs, each arranged in counters as in a jewelry store display. But perhaps because there wasn't an imminent danger from thieves, here the counters had no protective glass.

I tried to be nice.

But I couldn't help laughing. I've been around on too many Halloweens.

Dr. Ramirez was perplexed, and I hated to hurt his feelings. I kept explaining that it was wonderful what he was doing; but thanks a lot, I just didn't think so.

When Dr. Ramirez told me that only one out of ten people would ever know the difference, I thought, 'That's great. If I go to a 100-person party, pretty soon ten people will be standing in a corner saying, 'Carolyn Shuck's nose is plastic isn't it?'

I asked Dr. Ramirez if people wore these glue-on noses at night. He told me that one man wore his for four days and four nights straight. Now, boys, what do you suppose that man was up to?

Your Dad was even more flabbergasted by Dr. Lang's announcement than I was. He rushed down to the clinic and told Dr. Lang we wanted a second opinion.

Dr. Lang said he could give us the name of a good man in Kansas City and another in Salt Lake City. He didn't mention Dubuque.

Yesterday I zoomed over on a plane to see Dr. Davenport and he assured me that he could still do the forehead flap, encouraging me to do it right away, saying it would be no worse than what I'd been through.

He wasn't critical of Dr. Lang, just shook his head and said that his failure was due to lack of experience with my specific problem.

Oh my. Life is hard, life is earnest, but a rubber nose is not my goal. If this happened to an aging Carol Burnett, she wouldn't be left looking like this, and I sure as hell am not going to be, either.

If I ever get a rubber nose, kindly tell only your closest friends, but only the first nine of them.

Your educations may be all you'll ever get. The rest will probably be on the end of my nose.

Until spring break . . . Tally ho.

Much love from Carolyn G. Shuck, your Mother

In reply, I got a very supportive letter from John with a little humor thrown in. "If your nose runs and your feet smell, you're standing upside down." But his main message was that I should give it to Dr. Lang in *his* nose.

Ted didn't answer. "You didn't answer my letter," I said when we talked by phone.

"Well, I just didn't know what to say."

But actions speak louder than words. Later, when Ted was at home, he cheered me by offering to rebuild my nose himself.

I wasn't altogether sure he was kidding. When he was four or five, long before he could read directions, he assembled the most complicated of model airplanes and boats. One day he sat down at my sewing machine and, using no pattern or diagram except that in his own head, constructed a perfect, three-dimensional backpack.

Fortunately, we didn't have any ether in the house, not even a drop of demerol, so we decided to abandon the whole affair.

Ellen was so angry that she volunteered to go to the clinic to do battle. She could do it, too. It's a good thing she couldn't drive, or Dr. Lang would have had his hands full.

To say I was disappointed when Dr. Lang failed to repair my nose was like saying the Englishman was disappointed when the tiger devoured his wife.

All my life I'd heard about people who had regrets over things they should have done differently. I'd thought them ridiculous. I'd had no regrets. After an interesting career, I knew my marriage was happy, and we had three great kids.

Well, now I had regrets. In spades.

If only, if only, if *only* I'd kept the appointment with Dr. Davenport for the forehead flap.

Again, we vacationed in California. This time we looked at houses for sale, as we planned to move to the milder climate of La Jolla.

When my family was away from our apartment, I shut myself in the bathroom and yelled and screamed out my despair. I didn't beat my head against the wall, because I knew it would hurt. But once I clenched my fists and beat on my knees, then grabbed a bar of soap and threw it into the tub so hard it bounced back out. Whenever I felt heartache and/or tears coming, I got off by myself and let those tears fall.

I yelled at Dr. Lang.

I yelled at the clinic.

And I yelled at God. I knew He wouldn't mind my yelling at Him any more than if one of my children were severely hurt and yelled out in anger at me. These outbursts of pure rage helped a lot. For the rest of the day I could manage.

It wasn't that I'd been through a year of five worthless surgeries. Only one had been painful. But by now my whole face looked terrible. My cheeks were sunken. A furrow between my eyes gave me a constant frown. A year before I'd been wearing tape on my nose, but at least the rest of my face had been normal. Now I was still wearing tape on my nose, but my face was mutilated.

In our first interview, when Dr. Lang knew my cancer had been removed by chemosurgery, he'd expressed great confidence he'd be successful.

"I don't think you'll have a funny looking nose," he'd said.

Now, after an entire year of multiple surgeries, Dr. Lang told me he'd never successfully repaired chemosurgery wounds.

Now I had a funny looking nose *and* a funny looking face.

"If dermatologists had been alert earlier to your nose cancer," he'd said, "I could've easily removed the cancer and turned up a cheek flap with perfect results."

At this self-serving remark I exploded. "I'd been *seen* by the clinic's dermatology department. Just four months before Dr. Mohs operated, your own dermatology department merely cauterized my nose, and even then I had to call their attention to its crusting and bleeding. They also looked at my forehead and chin and did nothing. Nothing."

"Your skin's been irradiated. It makes it impossible to work with."

"What would you have done if the dermatology department *had* discovered the spreading cancers on my forehead and chin? If my skin is impossible to work with, how would you have repaired those areas after you removed the cancers?"

"Let's leave your forehead and chin out of this."

"Well, I'm happy to have them still a part of my face."

The reason for this debacle lay in lack of good judgment on the part of Dr. Lang and, alas, on my part.

Over that year of repeated surgery, I didn't once ask what is always THE ELEMENTARY QUESTION: "How many noses, defective like mine, have you reconstructed successfully?" Had I asked this question, Dr. Lang's answer would have been, "None." My horrendous experience should be an example to anyone seeking medical treatment: Go where they do *your specific treatment or repair every day*, and do it well.

The clinic has saved many lives. I know a person who would cross the country to go there for a tonsillectomy. Her confidence is based on her repeated good experience there. Some departments are renowned with good reason.

But no clinic or medical group can possibly be better for you than the specialist who is directly involved in your particular problem. The best specialist may well be practicing elsewhere.

Shortly after my fiasco at the clinic, it started sending serious skin cancer cases to Dr. Mohs. A more recent head of plastic surgery at the clinic said, "In his hands, Mohs' technique is nothing short of miraculous."

Incidentally, all names at the clinic are fictitious, including Dr. Lang's. I bear him no ill will. Certainly he had good intentions.

But I needed more than good intentions. I needed someone who could fix my nose.

8.

PLAIN
AS THE NOSE
ON YOUR FACE

The day after Dr. Lang's announcement that he could do nothing more, I flew to Madison to see Dr. Davenport. It had been almost a year since I'd wobbled out on limp legs to sign up for the forehead flap.

"Naturally," I said, when I saw Dr. Davenport, "I'm sick that I went to the clinic first."

"Don't feel too bad, Mrs. Shuck. Dr. Lang's good; he simply hasn't had experience repairing Mohs' wounds."

"But what'll I do now?"

"I can still do the forehead flap."

"Oh, what a relief. Do you really mean it?"

"Of course." He gently pinched my nose and ran his fingers over my forehead. "Sometimes we've used ear pieces to repair noses when the patient is squeamish about major surgery but they won't work in your case. You'd end up with a mosaic."

"When could we do it?"

"If I were you, I'd do it right away."

"You mean, hop right back on the horse?"

"Yes."

I breathed a sigh of relief and ran the back of my hand across my forehead. "I feel as if I've just come in on a life raft and landed on a safe shore."

Dr. Davenport smiled. "It won't be any worse than what you've been through; probably not as bad."

"You'll never know how grateful I am. I can't wait to go home and tell my husband."

"Isn't that terrific?" I said after I'd relayed my news to DeWitt.

"Carolyn, you can't have more surgery," he said, "the forehead flap could kill you." My feeling of deliverance disappeared like a plume of smoke in strong wind.

"That's silly." My stomach had turned suddenly sour. "Plastic surgery is only skin deep."

"Yes, but remember, there are four major operations within six weeks."

"You don't understand. I can't go on like this. I'm dying to have the forehead flap."

"It's not just me. The Narwolds are worried about you too. They called and told me they have a friend in Tulsa who wears a prosthetic nose. They say it's very good looking, even more attractive than her former nose."

"I'll bet."

"At least try one."

I knew that part of his resistance was due to the simple bad timing of it all. DeWitt had just resigned his position and we were planning a move to La Jolla. We were going to be very busy, selling our house, buying a new one in La Jolla, and entering Ellen in school there come fall.

"All right. I'll have a prosthesis made, to see if we can avoid any more surgery. But I haven't signed anything formal."

"Good. I'm sure it will all work out all right."

I knew this wasn't a move in the right direction, I just knew it. I was being forced to submit to the clinic's failure. That steel cage was being lowered over me again.

But for DeWitt, I could see how a prosthesis would be a happy ending from his point of view. And who knows? Maybe it could be a practical solution. With a bit of luck, it really could look like my former nose.

To get a first hand report, I phoned the Narwolds' Oklahoma friend.

"You don't know me, but I understand you're a friend of Marilyn and Lew's."

"Yes?"

"So am I. I've had a problem with skin cancer on my nose and they tell me you wear a prosthesis. They say it's very attractive."

"Not really."

"Marilyn and Lew told my husband they think it's even better looking than your former nose."

"They never saw my former nose."

"Well, do *you* like it?"

"No, not at all."

She sounded sad but could be just one more negative person, or maybe I got her on a bad day.

In April, I went to see Dr. Ramirez, the clinic's prosthesis maker.

He took an impression of my nose and face, using soft, clay-like material.

"I'll use this impression to make a plaster cast of your nose and face. Then I'll sculpture a wax nose cap, fitting it snugly over the plaster cast's nose.

Next, the wax nose cap will be duplicated in flexible plastic.

That'll be your prosthesis."

"You make it sound easy enough."

"Yes, It's a pretty ingenious procedure. From there I'll sculpture the nose cap to complement your face."

He showed me a piece of the flexible plastic material.

"It looks a lot like real skin."

"See here? Tiny blue and red blood vessels can be drawn in."

"It does look amazingly real." I hated to admit that it really did.

"Do you have a patient in Minneapolis who wears a prosthesis? A patient I could go see?"

He gave me the name of a woman who lived not far from our home.

That evening I phoned her. "Could I possibly come over right away to see your prosthesis?"

"Yes, but you'd better hurry if you want to get a good look. It's getting dark."

I rushed over and in the lamplight her prosthesis looked like a real nose.

"I'm a public health nurse," she said with a smile. "In two years no one has ever noticed I have a prosthesis." She seemed normally cheerful.

"I can see why. It looks very real to me."

"I think it's smart of you to get one rather than have more surgery. If you have more skin cancer, plastic surgeons may have to remove more of your nose. When they do, you can just have a larger prosthesis made. Much easier than to have to start all over with plastic surgery."

This wasn't one of my concerns. With Dr. Mohs' technique I was sure all my nose cancer had been removed. Even if anything new did sprout up he could get it while it was still tiny.

"Under my prosthesis, my whole nose is gone. Twice I've had

to have more cancerous tissue removed and each time the clinic's made me a larger prosthesis."

"Well, the clinic's certainly done a good job. You'd never know it wasn't your real nose."

I noticed she wore glasses. The frames hid the lines where the prosthesis is attached: across the bridge of her nose and down each side.

"You're wonderful to have let me barge in on you like this. Thank you so much. I'll tell Dr. Ramirez I saw you and congratulate him on the job he's done."

When I got home I told DeWitt all about her. "Honestly, with her glasses on, you'd probably never know. That's what Dr. Ramirez had suggested. That I wear glasses with clear lenses, so the frames could conceal the attachment of a full nose prostheses."

"I'd hate to see you wear glasses. They'd hide your eyes, and they're beautiful."

So, of course, I couldn't even consider wearing glasses.

The next day I called Dr. Ramirez and gave him the go ahead. "But I only want a partial prosthesis to cover the lower part of my nose, the part that's defective."

"All right, I'll get started right away."

When I hung up, I realized I was really looking forward to trying on my new plastic nose. Would I finally have a nose that looked like mine used to?

But when I tried it on, the following day, my stomach turned over. Dr. Ramirez could have modeled my prosthesis after Pinocchio's nose.

"I understand that the thin plastic has to enlarge my nose a little, because it has to fit over it. But why does it have to be so much *longer* than my original nose?"

"I think it's perfect. One of my best."

"My nose was never *this* long." Can't you make it a *little* shorter?"

"No."

"Why not?"

"I've worked very hard on it, and I'm not going to change it."

"Even if it would look at lot better to me?"

"I've told you, it's one of my best. I'm proud of it, and I'm not going to change it. Believe me, it's all psychological. It only looks long to you because you've had a snubbed off nose for a year."

I was sick. This was far worse than anything I'd endured during the surgeries.

Perhaps because he was predisposed to like Latin noses, he didn't know how to sculpture one becoming to my Swedish face. I could see that if I were ever to get Dr. Ramirez to make even a minor change, it would be an uphill battle.

So I decided to try to wear it.

Had my Pinocchio prosthesis been made of purple velvet encrusted with rubies and emeralds, it couldn't have seemed more conspicuous to me. When I'd first worn it around Minneapolis, I'd worn a piece of Micropore tape to cover part of it. I thought that when I left off the tape, others would think my surgery had been completed; that the prosthesis was my new, actual nose.

But in May, I attended a four-day regional meeting of women's clinics in Denver and decided to do it with a nude nose. It wasn't long before I noticed Minneapolis acquaintances looking at me curiously.

I pulled Barbara, one of my closer friends, aside. "Tell me, is it noticeable? Be honest."

"Well, you see, I know you're wearing it. To be perfectly honest, it looks to me like an ingeniously contoured flesh-colored bandage, shaped like a nose. Probably others will never notice."

An ingeniously contoured flesh-colored bandage, shaped like a nose? Oh God. My stomach churned, and for a moment, I thought I'd throw up.

But I knew I had to get used to the stares and my self-consciousness. For the rest of the day, I pretended to have a cold. I frequently took out a handkerchief and faked blowing my nose. But the Minneapolis contingent really started giving me curious looks.

Fortunately, Barbara and I shared a hotel room. We had a laugh over the whole awful thing. But if I fooled Barbara, I couldn't fool myself. I wasn't amused, not one bit.

I wondered how it would feel to jump from that window? No, I couldn't let myself think like that. Maybe it was good I was sharing my room. Alone, the way I felt, I might really have been tempted by oblivion.

On my way home, the conference over, I sat next to a member of the conference board. She and I were mere acquaintances, but I felt I had to pour out the truth to her. "Marge, I hope you won't mind my unburdening myself to you. I've felt awful throughout this conference. I'm wearing a nasal prosthesis and I absolutely despise it. You wouldn't believe how depressing it is for me."

"I'd heard you were wearing one. After all the surgery you've been through, I thought it was wonderful that they could make such things. It looks great to me."

I knew she was trying to make me feel better, but to me the shape was hideous.

It's true that beauty is in the eye of the beholder, but in this case I was the important one. After all, I was the one who had to look at it day after day in some mirror. Not Dr. Ramirez. My thoughts became increasingly bitter. After their dermatology and plastic surgery departments messed me up, you'd think the least the clinic could do is make a prosthesis I like. Besides, they're working with inert material, not real skin. I don't expect it to be exactly like my old nose, but it could be more that size and shape. It's as if I'm struggling with Dr. Ramirez to make me a blonde page-boy wig, the way I've always worn my hair. But he insists the auburn curls he's designed are far prettier.

I went to see my clinic internist, Dr. Morgan.

"Couldn't you please call Dr. Ramirez and tell him to make me a prosthesis that isn't so long? All I want is one that looks more like my old nose."

But Dr. Morgan wouldn't even look at me. Instead, he leafed through a periodical on his desk.

So much for the relaxed, friendly man I used to know. I got up to leave.

He jumped up, the magazine falling onto the floor. "No, no. Please stay, Mrs. Shuck. Now don't go away mad."

Was he worried I might bring charges against Dr. Lang or the clinic? God, what did he take me for, a damn fool? I knew that if I wanted any plastic surgeon to do more work, I couldn't afford to be known as a threatening patient, the type that might sue. I knew I had to appear calm and serene. *And I'd do it if it killed me.*

But I also knew that when things go sour at a large clinic, the patient has no advocate. I was a stain on their reputation, a conspicuous, visible stain. There was no hiding me. Now I was on the outside of an armed clinic castle surrounded by a moat, and all the drawbridges were raised. This enormous medical bureaucracy had become one unyielding monolith.

In early June, I decided to get a more suitable prosthesis made at another source. I went to a man who made the clinic's prosthetic material and had his manufacturing operation in what had been a barn in the countryside near a tiny Wisconsin hamlet. He'd made his own tiny nasal prosthesis and offered to work on one for me.

His office was in the kitchen of a large farmhouse close to the barn. He insisted I stay as a guest in a bedroom on the second floor of the farmhouse. To occupy myself, I read in a downstairs library. A secretary and bookkeeper worked in the kitchen office for only eight hours of the day. At night I was alone, and there were no locks on the doors. I'd always been uneasy staying alone in a city. Out in the country I was petrified.

For four days the same message from the barn was relayed every few hours through the secretary, over and over again.

"It'll be just a little longer, Mrs. Shuck."

It was an eerie rendition of everything I'd heard over the year at the clinic. "I'll need to do just a little more work on the right side, Mrs. Shuck." Then "I'll need to do just one more touch-up, Mrs. Shuck." Or "I need to do just a little more work on the tip, Mrs. Shuck."

"It'll just be a little longer, Mrs. Shuck."

The prosthesis my new-found friend produced was not at all satisfactory. After five days and nights with no one to talk to, I felt as though I'd been locked up in solitary for months. I'd allowed my hopes to rise, but the trip had proved worthless. Over the past two years I'd many times been angry, furious, shocked, even desperate. Now I was far more depressed than I'd ever been.

When I returned to our house I flew into DeWitt's arms. For the first time in front of him, I broke down and cried uncontrollably.

We'd bought a house in La Jolla, where Ellen would enter school in September. She and I were to fly to California in late July; DeWitt would stay behind until October to wind up business affairs. I held tight to his neck and buried my face in his chest. "I can't move to California and live there for three months without you. I just can't."

How I wanted him to hold me and tell me that he loved me

now and he'd always love me. That no matter what happened, I'd always be beautiful to him and that he couldn't bear to be away from me, either.

But few men have scripts in their hands for a scene like this. I'm sure he didn't know what to say. He gently pushed me away, fixed me a drink, and brought me up on the new details of our California move.

Our house sale had closed. The buyers were to move in on August 1. I'm sure DeWitt thought it would be impossible to rearrange our plans, and that I'd get over my little upset. He'd always seen me able to rebound quickly. Within half an hour after my outburst, he'd phoned the moving company to set a date to pick up our furniture, and had made airline reservations.

I was still a somewhat resilient tree, brought low in storms but ever still managing to right myself. But now rebounding required a lot of effort.

I couldn't help but wonder: did DeWitt still love me? More than schedules? More than the furniture?

I didn't want to enter California insecure with a crazy nose, and time for getting a suitable prosthesis was running out. It was the last of June.

I used fingernail scissors to snip away at the soft plastic tip of the Pinocchio prosthesis until it was down to the size of my old nose. To me, it looked a lot better.

The next day, I drove to the clinic to show Dr. Ramirez the changed prosthesis. I was determined he make me a new one, using the pared-down shape as a model.

"Good God, what have you done?"

"This is the size and shape I want."

"The one I made you was a work of art. I spent over two hours just sculpting the pattern. You have terrible taste. I told you before that I'm not going to change it, and that's that."

But I wouldn't give up. Two days later, I went back to see him.

I made it a point to stare at his two-tone shoes, never lifting my eyes.

"Don't you like my shoes?"

"It doesn't matter whether I like them or not. You like them, and you're the one who's wearing them."

Either I'd made my point, or Dr. Ramirez was sick of seeing me. He made a new prosthesis, shaped much like the one I'd pared down. At last, I thought it attractive. It should have been; it cost as much as a Porche.

The lower edges attached to the inside of my nostrils, blocking air. I asked Dr. Ramirez how I could blow my nose. He had no satisfactory answer, nor did he tell me how I could breathe without the open-mouthed expression of a child with adenoids.

A few days later, DeWitt and I went out. "Now people don't turn around to stare at you, Carolyn." It was meant to be comforting but wasn't. I'd been unaware of people's stares.

Unfortunately, a nasal prosthesis is worn in the middle of the face. If God had only placed the nose neatly behind the left ear.

But I pasted it on. Straight. And left for California.

9.

FEELINGS
ARE REAL

Prostheses do look real. But they simply are not. Gluing it on and blending it in to match my other makeup was no mean trick. At times, when I was about to drive the car pool, the adhesive would give way and one side would suddenly spring loose or wrinkle. And what would happen if I really had to blow my nose? What if the doorbell rang, the prosthesis still in a drawer? The first thing I did when I got up in the morning was to glue it on, but several times a day I'd press the edges against my nose, making sure it was secure, and even still there.

They also wear out quickly. I'd heard it was impossible to order a new one and get it sent out immediately so I bought several, enough to last at least a year, since I'd be living more than two thousand miles from the clinic.

Minneapolis friends alerted La Jolla friends, who spread out a welcome mat in fine and fancy fashion. On a weekend when DeWitt was in California, we were introduced at a large dinner dance. I stood in the receiving line the whole time wondering, is my prosthesis noticeable? Will it stay put? Fortunately there was plenty to distract attention—mine and others'—away from my nose. The lighting was dim, the guests seemed cordial and warm-hearted, the music was great for dancing, and drinks were flowing freely. And despite my worrying, my nose stayed glued on. It was a gala. I began to feel very much at home in La Jolla.

The next week's mail brought an invitation to a costume party, on an evening when DeWitt would be back in Minnesota.

"It's a Swiss Swing, whatever that is," I told DeWitt on the phone.

"Go. It'll do you good."

So I rounded up a waitress outfit from a German restaurant down the street and thought I looked pretty nifty, almost Swiss.

The night of the party, I sat outside in my parked car silently watching the well-lit and decorated house. I'd attended a lot of parties alone, but those were among old friends.

But I opened the door, straightened my dress, walked down the steep driveway, and greeted my hosts and fellow guests, all in Swiss costume. It was the wedding anniversary of two generations.

A costumed child followed me around the house while I was introducing myself and trying to be charming. She was small, probably about four, but her voice was that of an operatic soprano.

"What *happened* to your nose?"

"Well, you see, Sweetie, I was in a bad car accident."

"But what *happened?*" she asked, in ever increasing decibels.

"It was a horrible accident, our car rolled over and over," I whispered, then moved away. For that moment, I was glad we'd been in such an accident, but sorry we'd lived through it. I realized my invisible nose wasn't so invisible after all.

At that moment, a man entered, also in costume. He wore a false nose and mustache, attached to a pair of horn-rimmed glasses.

The stone in my stomach began to evaporate. I wanted to run

over and say, "Hi, Bud, I'm your partner for the evening." I didn't, but at least I knew the little soprano would have another nose to occupy her.

Most people I encountered over the years of trying to save my face were unusually kind. But when I wore the prosthesis, I was very sensitive.

Once, in a fabric store, a little boy came up to me and looked me straight in the eye. "Lady," he said, "you're ugly."

I went to my car and cried. I'd begun to lose perspective. Moving to another town, wearing a new plastic nose, was too much. My old confidantes were two thousand miles away. My new friends were kind and hospitable, but I felt that even the new, improved prosthesis was too conspicuous.

I could have endured it more easily if I'd been able to bring myself to tell people about it. But exactly how does one work a false nose into the conversation? They might not notice it on first meeting, especially if it was dusk and the light was behind me. And I didn't want to bring it up to people who didn't already suspect. But if the makeup had disguised it well enough, and the adhesive suddenly loosened, what then? Obviously, it would be a bit too late to bring up the subject.

I think I'd have been more comfortable if I could have worn a sign around my neck that read, "My nose is plastic."

Why I was so ashamed about something I had no control over, I'll never know. But for people who wear a prosthesis, it's a common feeling. A man who wears a tiny prosthesis on the side of his nose told me, "After two years, I still feel like people are eyeing it."

On our first Thanksgiving in La Jolla, Fame Bell came down from Palm Springs. We'd formerly lived in Keokuk. And after my arrival as a bride, Fame had been the most welcoming of DeWitt's friends.

She didn't like just anyone, but she liked the Shucks a lot. And if she liked you, there wasn't a more supportive friend. She fed your ego until it was bursting.

"Your whole family looks like they just stepped out of *Town and Country*," she once told me.

With my finger nails chipped? John and Ted as scrubby little boys? DeWitt driving an eight-year-old car? Of course she exaggerated. But I lapped it up, anyway, like a starved kitten at a bowl of cream.

I hadn't seen Fame since my face cancer began but we'd kept in touch. She knew I had a prosthesis and wasn't happy about it. She always gave me a big lift, and I couldn't wait to see her.

But when she got to our home, something in me started weeping. With my rubber nose and distorted face, I felt I'd toppled from the imaginary pedestal on which she'd put me. It was more difficult to face Fame, a long-time friend, than complete strangers.

She and Ellen were fighting over who'd make the mashed potatoes, when the phone rang. It was Barbara, with whom I'd shared the hotel room at the Denver convention.

"How are you *really* getting along, Carolyn?"

For a moment, I almost lied, but found I couldn't manage a trace of my old enthusiasm. "Every day I die a little," I told her.

Almost three months after Ellen and I moved to California, my new dermatologist found a malignancy. It was on my neck, exactly where I'd had another cancer removed ten years before. I called Dr. Mohs to report on the new man.

"I asked him, 'If you remove it, how will you know you've got it all out?' He told me, 'I've got fingers, I can feel; eyes, I can see.'"

"That's a poor way to delineate the extent of a skin cancer."

"Think I'd better come back there?"

"Yes."

"Let me see what I can do. I'll call you back."

I remembered what happened when other dermatologists removed skin cancers—they'd missed some, and the cancers continued to grow. That's what caused all my trouble.

I phoned DeWitt in Minneapolis. "I noticed a rough spot on my throat, so I went to a dermatologist here. It's in the same place where they removed a cancer about ten years ago. I've got to go back to Dr. Mohs."

"Can't someone there remove it?"

"No, not with any assurance. I've called Dr. Mohs; he thinks I should come to Madison."

The silence on the other end told me all I needed to know about his deep disapproval.

"I've got to go back. Frannie's offered to keep Ellen."

There was another long pause, then I heard him take a deep breath.

"If you feel you just have to."

After Dr. Mohs took out the small cancer, I went to see Dr. Davenport, the plastic surgeon.

"Your prosthesis is very good, one of the best I've seen. Maybe you're just not used to it yet."

"Oh, Dr. Davenport." My shoulder drooped, and I couldn't even look at him for fear I'd burst into tears.

"Do you want to know what my nurse says about you?"

"What?"

"Mrs. Shuck lights up the whole waiting room when she walks in."

Lights up the whole waiting room.

I clutched this wonderful compliment to my breast all the way back on the plane, but it warmed my heart for only two days. Soon my spirits drifted downward.

Only last January, Dr. Davenport urged me to do the forehead flap right away. What changed his mind? Was the prosthesis that good, perhaps better than a forehead flap might turn out? Or maybe he's had second thoughts about my irradiated skin? Oh, God.

DeWitt was in La Jolla for the weekend, and I confided my fears.

"I'm terribly confused about Dr. Davenport's change in attitude. I can't imagine what's happened. Maybe he thinks things are going to get even worse."

"Well, in August, I made a trip to see Dr. Mohs and Dr. Davenport. I told them I didn't want you to have more surgery."

"You *didn't.*"

"I don't want to see you go through any more suffering."

"But I'm suffering now."

DeWitt shook his head.

I knew he felt that way because he loved me. After all, how would I feel if he said, "Your deformed nose bothers me. For heaven's sake, Carolyn, do get it fixed?" I'd be crushed.

Still, I had to know whether DeWitt's visit was the reason Dr. Davenport praised the prosthesis, or if there was something else. I telephoned his office right away.

"I know about DeWitt's visit, and I know you said it looks great, but I'm getting very depressed wearing the prosthesis. Tell me, honestly, what would you do if you were in my place?"

He took a deep breath. "I'd have to do something."

"Why?"

"I couldn't get up every morning and paste that thing on."

At last his true view. What a relief to know my reaction wasn't abnormal.

It was all I could think about: how to have a nose with real, living skin. With maybe thirty years ahead of me, did I want to paste the prosthesis on two or three times a day and make it up? The surgery might take one or two years. But didn't a year or two of frustration and Micropore tape outweigh a possible thirty years of glue, makeup, and embarrassment?

"No." DeWitt said when I brought it up again. "No, I don't want you to have more surgery unless it's certain it will be successful."

But I knew no one could guarantee anything. And I also knew having the surgery would in effect put DeWitt through surgery too; he'd make the long trip back to Wisconsin with me. He'd always gone with me when I needed general anesthesia, and the forehead flap would be five surgeries over six weeks, with two more operations the next year.

I didn't know *what* to do. And indecision can cause anxiety, depression.

Something I couldn't allow myself to slip into. I knew I was a very fortunate woman despite my problems with skin cancer. After all, I was extremely lucky just to be alive with no brain damage and with normal eyesight. Maybe the best thing to do was to get busy helping others, count my blessings, and forget about my nose.

While living in Iowa, I'd spent fifty to seventy hours some weeks to see a women's health clinic through its birth pangs. From there, we organized satellites in neighboring counties. Thousands of families were helped. Immersed in seeing that poor women got care, I'd never have stopped for anything so minor as a new nose.

Wasn't there a vital project out here I could sink my teeth into?

I thought a lot about Lula. For seven years, she'd worked for DeWitt and me in Keokuk. She's the gingerbread baker that Ellen still loves; the woman John and Ted say has such a neat head.

DeWitt used to say, "Under other circumstances she could have headed U. S. Steel." She was so loaded with charisma, she could get people to do anything.

It was Lula who forced us to start the women's clinic. After it was set up, she wouldn't let me rest in the comfortable cocoon of my world. She drove me out of my home, up plank sidewalks, into homes where I'd find flies covering a newborn, or a mother frying flour and water cakes to feed her half-dozen children. She kept her aching foot in my back until we got every poor woman in the county to the new clinic.

"I've been pregnant ten times," Lula once told me.

"I find that hard to believe, you're so smart."

"Mrs. Shuck, people like me only know that people like you have some secret way of not getting pregnant."

After that, I was more determined than ever that our clinics succeed.

Even though she'd worked me so hard, I was as fond of Lula as were our children. Still, I was jealous that every party wound up in the kitchen, when I thought myself so entertaining; peeved, that friends consulted her privately, when I dispensed such good advice.

When we left Keokuk and moved to Minneapolis, Lula and I remained good friends. I encouraged her to get an education. She became a night telephone operator and took classes in the daytime at a neighboring small college. She got her B.A. degree, then her Master's, then finally a position as Head of Family Counseling of Northern Missouri. All this in spite of not attending a regular high school; completing her high school equivalency by taking a correspondence course.

How I longed to be back in the days when she worked for us, so that I could see her every day. Wearing the prosthesis, I'd gladly have paid her the standard psychotherapist fee just to talk a little cheer into me. She could sit on a chair while I scrubbed my own kitchen floor.

"A well-trained singer can warble right over a frog in her throat," a church soprano told me. "A great singer can throw her voice over a defect severe as acute laryngitis."

Lula's personality sang right over her "defect." Of course, her defect wasn't real; it existed only in the distorted, half-blind eye of society. But how visible and permanent it was. Lula was black.

My defect, the prosthesis, didn't prevent my children from attaining the topmost level in any field. But, even though things were changing, Lula's defect had curbed her children's progress.

If Lula could sing over her defect so effectively, why in God's Name couldn't I do the same? I felt helpless, trapped. I just couldn't bring myself to swallow the thought of living with the prosthesis. I even thought it hard to choke down food, and within weeks after gluing on the prosthesis, I'd lost ten pounds.

"Don't ever feel sorry for me if I die young," I said to Ellen one evening. "I really don't care about living too long."

"*Mother . . . .*"

"I'm sorry, I can't believe I've said such a thing. It's just been a bad day. I don't really feel that way."

I turned back to the book I was reading, but I was shocked that I'd voiced my fears to Ellen. Even to have such a thought was self-destructive. But I couldn't help myself thinking that way, and soon it got worse.

At the bottom of a hill, I'd have to put the car in park to keep from plunging into ongoing traffic. I had to push myself into the market, concentrate hard on what I had to buy to make for dinner. Force myself to cook those groceries and get a meal on the table.

A new friend invited me to lunch at her home. I made my best attempt at conversation but a fog kept closing in on me. I don't remember what we said and, for a moment, even drifted out of consciousness.

I needed help. Fast, while I could still realize I needed help.

At home, I called Louise Warren. Just after I'd arrived in California, I'd sat next to her at a luncheon and she'd told me she once used a psychiatrist who helped her a lot.

"Louise, I'm getting very depressed. Can you get me the name of a good psychiatrist or psychotherapist?"

"Sure. Go to Maria Bowen. She's terrific. She was a colleague of Carl Rogers. I'll find her phone number and call you right back."

"Thanks. You'll never know what you've done for me."

The week of my appointment, the hours dragged by. A heavy, heavy cloud hung over my head. When the day finally came, I drove about fifteen miles up the coast to a nearby seaside village. Dr. Bowen had given me good directions, and I quickly found the modest little bungalow where she saw clients.

Cautiously, I opened the unlocked outside door and stepped into a small, empty waiting room. On a counter were help-yourself makings for coffee or tea. I sat down in a wicker chair next to a small table littered with a variety of magazines. Dr. Bowen's name was on a closed door facing me. Other doctors' names were on two other closed doors.

Soon her door opened and a man came out, shut the door, nodded at me, and left through the door I'd come in.

In few minutes, her door opened again, and a tall woman with dark brown hair and friendly brown eyes came out.

"Carolyn Shuck?"

"Yes, I telephoned you."

"I'm Dr. Bowen." She reached out to take my hand. "Just call me Maria. Come in, won't you?"

"Your directions to get here were perfect."

"Good."

Her comfortable sandals, printed cotton skirt, and casual blouse made me feel at ease in my everyday shirt and slacks. She looked to be in her late thirties, possibly forty.

"Just have a seat on the sofa." She sat in a reclining chair, facing me, and shoved her footrest over so I could put my feet up.

"This is such a relief. You just don't know how depressed and confused I've been. But don't worry, I'm going to tell you."

"I want you to." She sat up straighter and leaned toward me on one elbow.

I took a deep breath and plunged in.

"I'm so mixed up I'm nearly insane. They had to remove most of the lower part of my nose because of skin cancer. Dr. Mohs—a skin cancer expert in Madison, Wisconsin, who did the surgery—he recommended this plastic surgeon in Madison, name's Davenport. Remember him. He proposed doing a forehead flap, which requires six surgeries, four anesthetics, and a stubble-covered skin tube. Really big stuff. Sounded so scary I went to a world-famous clinic for a second opinion. Their solution sounded a lot simpler, so I jumped right up on their operating table. Not just once, but *five* times."

"Hang on. This clinic proposed something different than Dr. Davenport?"

"That's right."

"Okay. Just wanted to get it all straight."

I took another deep breath and tried to slow down.

"After those five operations at the clinic, they said they couldn't do another thing and made me this plastic nose after I insulted the doctor's shoes. I've got it pasted on now. I hate the thing. Sometimes I think if I have to get up one more morning and paste it on, I'll go absolutely crazy. Last January, when I went back to Dr.

Davenport, the man in Madison who's done so many of Dr. Mohs' repairs—this was before I had the prosthesis made—I remember his *exact* words; in fact, they haunt me now. He said, 'I can still do the forehead flap. If I were you, I'd have it done right away. It won't be any worse than what you've been through. Probably not as bad.' But my husband, DeWitt, was retiring and we were moving to La Jolla, so DeWitt pretty much insisted I have this plastic nose cover made."

"And how do you feel about that?"

"I'm dying to have Dr. Davenport do the forehead flap. After going through so much plastic surgery, I know it isn't painful. It's only skin deep."

I hit the arm of the sofa. "I should have gone to Dr. Davenport in the beginning, it just gnaws at me that I didn't. But at least he's still willing to do it. The big opposition is coming from my husband, DeWitt."

"Sounds like you've been through quite an ordeal."

"I suppose nothing's as good or as bad as it sounds. I just want to finish what I started to do; get my nose repaired. But now I'm stymied, blocked."

"By DeWitt?"

"Yes. You know what *really* burns me up? Before he made his final move to California this last October, he made a secret trip to Madison to see both Dr. Mohs and Dr. Davenport, he told them *he* didn't want me to have any more surgery. I think it was all part of his winding up his business affairs in Minnesota before he came to La Jolla in October. Every year he makes up a yearly budget on a large yellow ledger sheet. One item is medical expense not covered by our medical insurance. I'm sure he thought he could get that item off his ledger sheet for good, if I'd just get the prosthesis and learn to accept it.

"DeWitt didn't go with me to hear Dr. Davenport's original proposal for reconstruction. He didn't go with me to that great clinic to hear their proposal for what was supposed to be a simple surgery. And after the clinic said they couldn't do anything more, he didn't go with me to hear Dr. Davenport tell me he could still do the forehead flap. He was perfectly comfortable letting me make all the decisions about my face.

"*Now* he's closed out all my options. I'm sure he told Dr. Mohs and Dr. Davenport, 'She's my wife and I'm taking charge of her face. I'll tell you what I want done.' But just whose nose is it, anyway?"

"You tell me."

"He doesn't even know all the options that are out there. I'm sure he thinks, 'She's all fixed up with a paste-on nose, so she has no room to complain.' How I feel about it isn't important."

"Did you *ask* him to go with you to hear these proposals for rebuilding your nose?"

"No."

"Can you afford more surgery?"

"Easily. We have wonderful medical insurance, and plastic surgery is far less expensive in the midwest than it is in California."

"Is it possible DeWitt's frightened? After all, you've already been through five surgeries."

We talked on a while about DeWitt, until Maria said,

"I hate to stop, but our hour is up and I have another client waiting."

Damn. And just as I was really getting going, too. I eagerly made another appointment.

On my drive home I felt a lot better. I'd gotten rid of a lot that had been festering inside me for a long time, more than I'd known was there. And I thought of what Dr. Bowen had said about DeWitt being frightened.

Frightened? DeWitt?

I thought about DeWitt growing up as the son of a country doctor. As a child, he probably heard a good deal of talk about people "going under the knife," and probably a lot about people dying in surgery.

I remembered all those times DeWitt had been with me before an operation where I'd be put to sleep. Because he knew I was dreadfully afraid of anesthetics, he'd stay with me as long as possible, walking alongside the gurney through the halls, into the elevator, again through more halls until he'd lean over to gently kiss me goodbye as they closed the doors between us when I entered surgery.

After the second operation at the clinic he'd kept a vigil in my hospital room long after darkness fell.

"I hated to leave you last night," he told me the next morning, "you looked so pale."

All this time, I thought I was the only one afraid I wouldn't wake up to see my "Dahlquist" sign, but the surgeries might have been much harder for DeWitt than for me. If the thought of a blood pressure check made his hands perspire, the anxiety from the thought of my further surgery must be heart- wrenching. Perhaps he felt he could endure no more suffering.

One time, we were having our lunch together in a hospital cafeteria, when, for no apparent reason, he'd shuddered.

"What's the matter?" I asked.

"I cannot *stand* hospitals."

I thought of how much DeWitt had already endured, and how much I loved him. Adored him, really. He was in a class by himself, and what integrity. In all the years I'd lived with him I'd never once seen him do an underhanded thing. Why in the world had I suspected him now?

DeWitt's biggest concern about my having the forehead flap had nothing to do with money. The thought of the surgery was probably very frightening to him.

On my next visit to see Dr. Bowen, I quickly sat down and started right in.

"I think you were right about DeWitt's being frightened about further surgery. He's really a wonderful man and I feel it was unjust to say what I did about him."

"I'm sure he is, but it's impossible to live in a close relationship and not ever have any mixed feelings. You were depressed, and many times depression is anger turned inward. Be sure to say anything you're thinking or feeling. Don't hold anything back. It's the only way you can work your way to a state of mind that will allow you to come to a clear decision."

I only went only four or five times to this excellent therapist, to sift out my thoughts and feelings. I did most of the talking during each session; Dr Bowen said little. But after each appointment I came away with something she *had* said to think about. She had an uncanny way of saying just the right thing at the right time. She also managed to keep my evaluations logical, whenever my thinking seemed to be sliding off track. Never did she tell me what to do, or even hint at what she might do under similar circumstances.

The whole process helped me to climb out of the pit I'd dug for myself. It was a lot like what my father did for me when I was stranded in that tar paper shack. He didn't tell me what to do and how to do it, he merely showed me the way out.

It's a normal desire to have one's own flesh, if possible, and with Dr. Bowen's help I made sure I'd be having further surgery for valid reasons, not to prove Dr. Lang wrong, and not because I felt DeWitt was making a decision that should be mine.

At home I talked with DeWitt. "I can't go on wearing the

prosthesis when there are other options available. If surgery is unsuccessful, then I can adjust to the inevitable and go back to a prosthesis."

"I was so worried about your reaction to the clinic's failure, I didn't want you to be disappointed again. I've been terribly depressed myself. I didn't know what to say, so I said as little as possible."

"I know how you hate hospitals. But can you help me now?"

"Of course. I want you to be happy."

Boy, how I'd waited to hear that. Finally, I'd decided.

I would take another go at having my own nose. Feelings are real.

10.

BACK ON
TRACK

I f I was going to be stuck in a hospital for six weeks, it would be
far more convenient to have my nose repaired near home.
California is teeming with plastic surgeons; some are famous for
rebuilding movie star's faces, mangled in accidents. In the spring of
1973, I combed the West Coast and consulted several doctors.

All politely declined the job.

One eminent surgeon, about to retire, showed me a schematic
diagram of the forehead flap. "This is the only way to go and it's
not a dangerous operation," he said. "But if you decide to have it
done, don't discuss it with your family; don't discuss it with friends.
Discuss it only with a plastic surgeon."

I must have looked puzzled because he put down the diagram.

"Trust me," he said, looking me right in the eye. "They'll think
it's butchery plain and simple. They won't believe anyone could
come out of it looking normal and will say anything to discourage
you from getting it."

I could understand that. I could hardly believe it myself.

"I wouldn't touch you. I rarely see a similar case in a year," another surgeon said, "but do get it done. People are enthusiastic about prostheses at first. Then they start leaving them in dresser drawers."

"Do you know anyone in California who could do it?"

"No. Go back to Davenport. He's done hundreds, probably thousands."

That May, on our way to John's Amherst graduation, DeWitt and I stopped in Madison.

"You know," Dr. Davenport said, "There's a good chance I can repair it by using pieces of your ears."

Whoa, hold up here. Has DeWitt's private visit colored his thinking? Just after the clinic failure, he'd mentioned earpieces, but said I'd end up with a mosaic.

"Dr. Davenport, I'm no longer afraid of the forehead flap."

"Oh, I realize that, but your tissues have softened a lot during the year-and-a-half since the clinic's last surgery. So much so that earpiece surgeries are a good possibility."

"Just what are they?"

"Composite grafts, minor surgeries. We'd do one every six months. It's an iffy procedure but I've had good luck with it. You'll have to keep your fingers crossed."

Suddenly, I could see myself running the three blocks from our house to the beach, hurling my box of prostheses far out into the Pacific to wash up on some distant shore. I could just imagine the puzzled look on the person's face who found it. My fears disappeared. After all, DeWitt couldn't object to these minor surgeries.

"Not to worry, Dr Davenport." I said, staring him straight in the face with my scarred, notched button-of-a-nose, and facial distortions. "I've always been a very lucky person."

He looked a little startled, but that's the way I felt. I didn't smother him with kisses or weep with joy, but I wanted to.

The word spread that I was taking another shot at having a nose, and friends did what they could to help. Catholics offered masses, TM friends meditated, Protestant and Jewish friends sent prayers floating upward.

Our children claim I've brought them up on voodoo and they refuse to practice it. But I continued working my superstitions. Why take chances when things are so precarious? Nightly, I wished on the first star, looked at three others before glancing back at the first. I kissed my upturned dress hems and wished on white horses, even those on billboards.

Whom was I fooling? All superstitious acts are primitive prayers.

But I also readied myself physically and mentally. I took mammoth doses of Vitamins C and E, and I made a THINK PINK sign to hang in my hospital room. Maybe my nose graft would read it, obey it, and become rosy-red, as required.

And I had the Twenty-third Psalm down pat.

When the tip is gone and part of the side is missing, rebuilding the nose isn't easy. I'd found that out the hard way. You need to grow enough skin onto the nose to build into the shape you want. Since the nose has a lining, the graft must first be lined with other skin. All skin must come from the patient's own body, or it will be rejected. When enough skin has been added it can be rearranged and shaped into a nose.

Because my skin is thin and had been X-rayed, the chore was unusually difficult.

The plan was to have three pieces from my ears grafted to my nose, one every six months. After a year I'd have enough ear tissue on my nose; then it would have to soften for six months before it could be rearranged and shaped, also in six month intervals. All told, it would take two-and-a-half years.

Finally, in July, nose repair got under way.

"The part of the ear we'll use is above the lobe where the edge of the ear is stiff with cartilage," Dr. Davenport said. "We'll take out a pie-shaped wedge."

"Will my ear be deformed?"

"Not noticeably. Since both sides of the wedge are covered with skin, it'll have its own ready-made lining."

"You see?" he pinched my ear gently, and wiggled it back and forth,

"It contains cartilage. That'll add stiffening. However, there's one big hitch. The wedge has to grow onto the nose with no blood supply feeding it, so the take isn't certain. To keep your nose from rejecting the graft, icy compresses will be applied for several days."

"Won't it hurt to have my nose packed in ice that long?"

"It won't be packed in ice. Icy compresses are gauze squares, dipped in ice water. For four days and nights, they'll be laid lightly over your nose graft every fifteen minutes. They'll be soothing, but you may suffer sleep loss."

It was a small price to pay.

I'd had all the shots that dry up secretions and paralyze the brain. As I lay on a gurney in the operating room, ready for the first surgery, someone told Dr. Davenport the anesthesiologist would be an hour late. Exasperated, he told a young Chinese resident to keep me company. Or was it to check my blood pressure? I didn't want to ask whether he was going to use acupuncture for anesthesia even though it was foremost on my fuzzy mind.

Despite the delay, the first surgery went perfectly. Dr. Davenport even took out the furrow between my eyes, so I didn't wear a frown. After a-year-and-a-half, my expression was back to normal, something Dr. Lang hadn't accomplished in three simple surgeries.

The gauze squares were supposed to be laid on the earpiece every fifteen minutes night and day, but the night nurses were letting them dry out. So I rang for an orderly.

"If you'll make it your personal duty to keep track of the time and see that these wet compresses are changed every fifteen minutes, I'll privately pay you ten dollars extra for your shift. Then, if you tell your replacement to do the same thing, I'll make the same arrangement with him. It's extremely important to me that this nose graft take."

For DeWitt, the trip couldn't have been exciting. He walked miles around the town, and became familiar with every street, shop, office, apartment, and university building. Today, I'm sure he could be a taxi driver in Madison with no map to guide him.

On Sunday, I did my own hiking and trotted clear across the hospital in my best robe to attend a service and offer thanks. After I sat down, I realized it was a Catholic mass.

I hoped no one could read my mind and know I started those birth control clinics. The priest turned around—he was very young—and I couldn't keep back tears while I smiled at him. He reminded me of the young priest who helped so much behind the scenes to start our first clinic.

At the ending of the mass, we sang the same song that closed our Presbyterian service in La Jolla.

> Love I leave with you, my friends,
> Agape love in all you do;
> Love I leave with you, my friends;
> I give to you so you can give to others too.

In our church at La Jolla, a thousand voices join a heavenly choir and magnificent pipe organ to send it soaring through the sanctuary. That morning, a tinny little tape recording accompanied about fifteen people, but never had that song sounded so beautiful.

In hospitals, great roommates are hard to come by. But when I got Reno, I hit the jackpot. With a name like that, what else could you expect?

"Why are you here?" I asked.

"Well, a year ago I had the hearing corrected in my left ear. Now it's my right ear's turn."

"It's wonderful they can do that. Is it a serious operation?"

"No. I'm just here overnight. Although I'm not sure it's so wonderful."

"Why not?"

"I have three boys, five, four, and two. With the noise level at my house, it would be more sensible to turn *down* the decibels. I should be buying some ear plugs at the drug store for my good ear instead of fixing the bad one."

"Why don't you wait till your boys go off to college?"

"I was tempted by the peaceful vacation I'd have here. Besides, my husband decides everything. He's a real macho type."

"My two boys were only thirteen months apart. When they were little, all I wanted for Christmas was a room at the Hotel Iowa for an hour each afternoon, away from the bedlam. I'd promise not to mess up the bed, just bring my own blanket and lie on top of the covers for a much-needed nap."

"Did you ever get that Christmas present?"

"No, but I wore ear plugs for a long time. I know just what you mean about your surgery being an unwise move. Maybe it won't be successful."

"I can dream."

They gave Reno a sleeping pill that first evening. "Oh, no," she said as she dozed off, "Now my vacation's almost over."

Her holiday ended when they released her the next morning. Dressed to leave, she was reluctant to go. She sat on the side of her bed for almost two hours and dallied over her goodbye lunch.

"I've had the nicest Fourth of July in my whole life, right here in this hospital room."

"Will someone help you out at home until you fully recover?"

"Oh yes," she said, "My helpless husband, his mother, his aging aunt who's an invalid, and of course my three rowdy boys."

The next week, a note came from Reno. "Someday I will be forced to commit a crime that will land me in jail, where my loved ones cannot get at me."

How I wished Reno had just one more ear so we could have scheduled twin surgeries.

One evening, during the first earpiece surgery, Rachel came to see me. I got a great lift from knowing that Dr. Mohs' nurse cared about me. She introduced her husband, John. It was then about seven-thirty and I knew Rachel had been working since seven in the morning.

"Oh, Rachel, am I ever glad to see you. Only this morning, I was thinking, it's been three years since you said that if anyone in the world could fix my nose, Dr. Davenport could." I looked at John, "You'd think she'd wash her hands of a dummy like me who went to the clinic instead."

"Of course she wouldn't." He winked.

Rachel smiled. "The important thing is, you're here now."

"I know this is a stupid question. You know I want a real-skin nose, not a prosthesis. But will Dr. Davenport's reconstruction be as attractive as my prosthesis was?"

She looked surprised. "Why, yes, they usually are."

John added: "You wouldn't believe some of the things he's done. I've seen amazing reconstructions of noses, lips, anything Dr.

Mohs has had to destroy. I think you'll be pleased."

I expressed my relief. "This is so encouraging!"

Rachel explained: "You ears will be shortened a little. Clip-on earrings may slip off, so before your next surgery, ask Dr. Davenport if he'll pierce your ears."

"Good idea," I said. Rachel had the answer for everything.

"We're on our way out to get a bite to eat, but let me know if you need anything," Rachel said reassuringly.

My voice almost broke. "You don't know how I appreciate your stopping to see me."

"We'll try to come in again before you leave." They spoke with one voice.

What wonderful people! Didn't they have a private life?

In the end, everything turned out splendidly. The first graft attached itself, partially filling the notch on the right side. My nose looked like a misshapen strawberry, but I knew the first step to getting enough skin on had been successful. I was in heaven.

Each time I entered the hospital I was optimistic, knowing I was that much closer to my new nose. But one nurse, a fixture, became my nemesis. She must have taken a special course in "Depressing the Patient with Facial Disfigurement." When I was about to delve into a book I was savoring, or ready to turn on the TV, in she'd come with a hang-dog look on her face, her large brown eyes misting. Somehow, she looked familiar, a lot like someone I know. Now who could it be?

Then she spoke. "You must have cried a lot of tears over your nose."

"I've shed a few tears, but my life in the outside world is really quite pleasant."

It was impossible to cheer her up. She refused to believe me.

Then I had it. She was the image of our neighborhood basset

hound, Solomon. From now on, she'd be Nurse Basset to me. I just hoped I wouldn't slip up and call her that.

Soon after I got home, I saw a casual male acquaintance at the market. I'd feared that people thought that under the prosthesis my whole nose was missing, so I felt compelled to show this man I had a real nose—no matter how tiny, misshapen, and bandaged. Since I only knew him slightly, he must have been surprised when I rushed over to greet him. Later I had to laugh. If he'd previously believed my plastic nose was real, he must have thought I'd wandered into a standing electric fan.

Well, I wouldn't have to put up with it for much longer. My nose would be completed in the spring of 1976. That is, if all went well.

But of course it would.

11.

GREEN PASTURES

E ventually, three pieces of my ears would be grafted to my nose.
But the surgeries were only small islands in an ocean of time,
quickly forgotten when I reentered California.

I probably looked more attractive when I was wearing the
prosthesis, but I didn't care. This was *my* nose, and I knew the
defects—covered once again with Micropore tape—were only
temporary.

I grew to love living in La Jolla, a town of only thirty thousand.
Most of the population had come from other parts of the country,
drawn to its oceanfront charm and year-round fine climate. There
were more stimulating, enjoyable people than I could ever get to
know.

There was Julia, for instance, always just returned from a trip
to some obscure spot on the globe. She'd tell me about it when we'd
have lunch at La Valencia. And fill me in on her Egyptian history
course at the university.

And Jeannie, that rarity, a native San Diegan. I'd cross the
border with her, and spend a Tijuana morning foraging for baskets,

baubles, and jalapeno peppers for her jelly; then wash down a Mexican lunch with margaritas.

Louise had written best sellers; three became movies. At eight years of age, she'd lost a leg. Her parents—certain she'd never marry—sacrificed to send her to college so she could earn her own living. Now she'd just married her fourth husband. I'd meet her for lunch every week at The Inn at Rancho Santa Fe. Constantly interrupting each other, we'd talk a-mile-a-minute for two hours. Driving home, I'd think of things I'd meant to ask her, tell her. I'd walk in the door and she'd telephone, also needing to wind up loose ends.

When we arrived in California, Bunty and Ed had taken us in, kids and all. When I was in Madison, I'd receive a letter from Bunty every day. They'd have us over for dinner the day we came home.

And Jimmie Jacques. Her upperclass Eastern breeding was as apparent as her down-to-earth sense. A Wellesley graduate, she'd been a head buyer at Macy's and a Hattie Carnegie model. Then she'd worked alongside her husband raising Hereford cattle and quarterhorses on their Wyoming dude ranch. She remembered those ranching days as glorious.

Jane and John had rescued me at the Swiss Swing party. Surprisingly, we'd found that my mother and John's father had both been in the Class of 1910 at Nebraska U. Both Jane and John were gifted with spectacular wit. Just looking at John, I couldn't help but smile. I knew he was getting ready to say something to make me laugh.

"I simply cannot believe in the doctrine of original sin," I once said.

"Well, if you're going to do a little sinning, it should be original to make it worthwhile." That was John.

I'd been asked to join another sewing club that didn't sew. All of the women had histories full of interesting surprises. In 1932, one had done the unheard of. A southern belle, she had flown unescorted to Shanghai to marry a famed aviator. Another had painstakingly raised an awkward, small, grey yearling to win the Kentucky Derby.

This sewing circle didn't specialize in luncheons like my Minneapolis cronies, but in stock market investing. Each month they met mid-afternoon, for a two-hour spirited discussion of hot tips from secret sources. They bought and sold with abandon, an activity that broke into a mad scramble just before five, when the husbands would arrive for drinks and dinner.

Once more, just as in Minneapolis, my defective nose was no barrier to with an invitation to join a delightful group.

Not only were our friends enjoyable, the shopkeepers were as well. In the building supplies store, clerks joked around in back of the counter. Their levity made me free to exchange a few quips of my own.

When I'd shop for a dress, my favorite salesperson didn't insist the number I tried on was becoming. Instead, we'd laugh together over how awful it was.

I took alterations to Elgin de la Hunte. A large woman, with lots of spare poundage (she was always asking me if I wanted to borrow some), she was invariably in high spirits. Her sewing-room-parlor, at most ten by twelve feet, overflowed with a clutter of books, art objects, and trailing plants, amidst all her sewing paraphernalia.

This artistic chaos had been acquired over years of rummaging through garage sales and secondhand stores, but chosen with discriminating taste. As soon as you walked into the topsy-turvy little room, right away you knew an intellectual, cultured person lived there.

She never walked, but somehow managed to run in this tiny, crowded room. As quick-witted as she was sure-footed, her fifteen-minute appointments could easily extend to forty-five. A book must be discussed, a world problem thrashed out, or a comical happening in the news related.

I imagined how different her life might have been if only some forebear had struck it rich. I could see her in a Paris salon, presiding over artists, writers, and connoisseurs of all the arts.

My freedom from former pressures also made life wonderful. DeWitt gave his time to four philanthropies. I was on sabbatical. Occasionally I'd compose a letter to the editor that I felt had impact. I'd attend the nominating committee meeting for the local women's clinic, but I'd resigned from the board. I was slothful and liked it.

When I'd go to Madison to see Dr. Mohs for small cancer removals, I didn't have to plan menus, shop for groceries, and cook meals in advance; I could just step on the plane. Ellen was now an independent fifteen. She and DeWitt could go out for Chinese, or she could cook her scrumptious fried chicken.

Life was far more relaxed with our children grown up. Back then days were tightly organized, not a minute wasted. Now clerks at the neighborhood market teased me about making three trips to get ingredients for a single recipe.

And could that be the same DeWitt who'd gone with me to Madison as bodyguard and sat stiffly erect in Dr. Mohs' hallway, his head in the *Wall Street Journal*?

Now he ran around at parties, kissing the ladies hello. He wore slacks embroidered with whales; navy cords adorned with yellow tees and golf balls.

Once, I looked twice at them. "You think those are golfer's slacks?"

"Aren't they?"

"Look closely. Those are yellow screws piercing white baseballs. They're slacks for screwballs." His buddies might tease him, but he continued to wear them.

And could this be the same closed, quiet, uncommunicative DeWitt who was yammering away, not letting me get one word in? I couldn't have been more delighted.

His surface change was a reflection of an inner change. He had time to let his interests expand. As President of the Art Museum, he broadened his interest in the arts; as Chairman of Scripps Clinic, he deepened his concern with medical research. Exposed to every segment of the community, as a member of the Parker Foundation Board, he was keenly aware of those less fortunate.

I'd taken up bridge, along with Planned Parenthood and family activities. No longer was bridge something to do with my hands as I talked. Bidding was learning to talk with your partner in a foreign language. Fascinating. Would I ever master it?

My days weren't long enough to enjoy the smörgåsbord of life spread before me. My life became as easy going and rich with pleasure as it had been long ago in Oklahoma. I'd stepped back to life as it was supposed to be. I'd come home.

"If, in another life," I said to Jane one day, "I could choose to come back to earth in any time period, to any place, be any person, I'd choose to come back right now to La Jolla as myself. I'd be living with DeWitt, know the same people, and have time to savor more of my present life."

It didn't enter my mind to say I'd come back with a perfect nose. Enough skin had been grafted. Soon it would be shaped.

Naturally, my nose was going to be great.

12.

SHOWERS OF BASAL CELLS

E ven while I was settling back into the idyllic life, new basal cell skin cancers kept cropping up with maddening frequency. When Dr. David Peters, the excellent dermatologist I'd found in La Jolla, first biopsied something on my face that turned out to be malignant, I asked,

"If you removed it, would you know you'd got it all out?"

He shook his head. "Go to Mohs."

Over the course of the following year, Dr. Peters pared off suspicious spots and sent them to a local lab. If they tested malignant, I'd fly back to Dr. Mohs. In 1973, I made ten trips to Madison. Each time he'd remove two or three cancers.

"These things seem to be raining on me," I said on one such visit.

Dr. Mohs shrugged. "It sometimes happens."

Patients waiting for Dr. Mohs are a little fraternity of kindred souls—after all, if you had that many gall bladder patients in one spot, just imagine all they'd find to talk about. Cream, and—oh, yes—lamb fat, and Vitamin E, and does it dissolve fat, and about one woman from Evansville who ate nothing but crushed apricot pits and never had one bit more gall bladder trouble. Imagine the chatter.

I got all sorts of tips from "honorary degree" doctors sitting in his anteroom. "Castor oil is a cure-all for skin cancer," one told me.

"Where should I put it? Inside or out?"

"Oh, just rub it on any suspicious spot."

Then why was she sitting there all bandaged up, just as I was?

Another one of these "doctors" leaned over to me and said, "Don't you believe all the nonsense you hear in this place. If you go home and stay home, all wounds uncovered, you'll heal a lot faster."

Before I took the plunge, I imagined that married life gave you unlimited time to lounge about, eat bonbons, and read murder mysteries. I was miffed at married women who crowded New York City busses during rush hour when I, a working woman, had to use them. They should have been home, eating their candies.

But married life didn't turn out that way. Within two years we had both John and Ted, and parenting shot the bonbon deal.

But now, when I'd return from Dr. Mohs' place, I was finally going to enjoy that married life. I had the bonbons in the house, and juicy literature on my bedside table. I'd uncover my wounds, daub them with mercurochrome—DeWitt had suggested a coordinating robe, beige with red polka dots—but then the telephone would ring.

"Oh, I look just too awful to go out."

"We don't care one bit."

"Give me forty-five minutes."

I never have been able to enjoy married life in the way I had imagined.

In March of 1974, a tiny place on my right cheek proved malignant. I called Dr. Mohs.

"The offices are being remodeled. Sorry, he isn't here. You might want to see Dr. Brown in Encino, California."

"Does he use the Mohs method?" I tried not to panic.

"He's been trained by Dr. Mohs. I'll get you his phone number."

I called Dr. Brown.

"I'm Mrs. Shuck. I've been a patient of Dr. Mohs and I need to have a skin cancer removed. Can you take care of me?"

"You'll have to come on Monday. It's the only day I practice chemosurgery. On other days I do routine dermatology."

"How about next Monday?"

"Come at nine in the morning."

On Sunday evening, DeWitt and I drove to Encino, three hours away. "It's wonderful this doctor's so close," I said.

"It's certainly more convenient than Madison. Maybe he'll be the answer, and you won't have to go to Madison, once your nose is finished."

The next morning, Dr. Brown cut and scraped—with no microscope examination—for what seemed fifteen minutes.

I didn't understand. Dr. Mohs always pared off a little slice and then examined it before he removed any more.

"How do you know all you are cutting out is cancerous?"

"The tissue is soft and mushy. I can tell."

Finished, his excavation was the size of a quarter and deep as the bowl of a teaspoon.

"Wait for the pathology report. I'm sending it over to the lab."

After a long two hours, the lab report came back. "I've removed all the cancer," he said. "I undermined all the margins, too, so I'm sure the report's correct. Too bad it's so large."

He filled the wound with a white, gooey paste that burned a lot.

"Want to get some lunch at the place down the street?" DeWitt asked.

"No. I want to put a good hour between that man's office and my bowl of soup."

God, this was scary. When I'd first seen the blemish in my magnifying mirror the week before, it was only the size of a pinhead. Was that pinhead blemish just the tip of a much larger underground cancer? My forehead, chin, nose, and now my right cheek, had produced large, spreading cancers. Where would it stop? What could I expect next?

That evening we went to a party.

"I saw the bandage on your cheek," a friend said the next morning. "Your eyes were big as saucers. You didn't say two words all evening." I appreciated her concern. But she didn't know the half of it. I was paralyzed with fear.

I phoned Rachel in Madison. "I hate to bother you, especially at home. I've leaned on you so much, it's a wonder you're still standing up. But I have to tell you what happened." I described the Encino experience.

"Well, it is true that soft mushy tissue usually indicates cancer. Without a lab in his office he probably wanted to get it all in one cutting," Rachel said.

"After this, I'll come back to you."

I was lucky I could make these trips without a major change in our lifestyle. But I wondered—what if another economic depression came?

"DeWitt, what would happen if our finances started to slide? Say, a depression hits?"

"We could always move to Madison."

I could tell he didn't think a depression was imminent, but thank heaven he was concerned enough about my skin to give it priority.

I trekked to Madison on the day after Thanksgiving, and again on New Year's Eve.

"Could we please arrange to die on the same day?" I asked Dr. Mohs, "With my skin, I don't want to outlive you."

"Perhaps we can concoct a mutual suicide pact," he said, without even looking up from his work.

But from my first visit to Dr. Mohs, I found him a sneaky man. My guess was that if my time came first, he'd just keep whittling away. And if he went before me, I doubted he'd stop by California to pick up an extra passenger.

As it turned out, this wasn't a shower of basal cell skin cancers. I was in a downpour.

13.

MOURNING AND CELEBRATION

I n August of 1974, more than four years after my serious skin
cancer bout began, success was at last in sight. In a few months
Dr. Davenport planned to start shaping my nose.

But on a certain beautiful day in La Jolla, Dr. Peters removed
a tiny piece of skin from the bridge of my nose, and it tested positive for cancer. Now more skin would have to be taken from my
nose, the nose that had been through nine reconstructions. I could
only pray that it would be only a small piece, and that the place
would heal over quickly. It just *couldn't* be the tip of a larger underground cancer like the one on my cheek. If it was, it meant more
skin grafting.

The day he found the cancer was one of those fairyland days in
La Jolla. The air seems to sparkle there as it does in no other place.
Through broad open doors, I looked out on our garden, a heavenly
oasis.

Tall eugenia hedges and eucalyptus trees enclose the spacious
brick patio and sunken lawn, making it private and secluded.
Flowering pear trees, which burst forth in the spring like white

popcorn trees, are lush and green year-round, along with the lime and lemon trees, the grape ivy, and all the other thriving foliage.

It was my green pasture. It restored my soul. But now my heart was like lead.

I called Dr. Mohs for an appointment, and was upset to find him on a rare vacation, not due back for a month. Instead, I cried on Rachel's shoulder.

"I wouldn't worry too much," she said. "A basal cell carcinoma normally grows slowly, not more than a millimeter a month."

"How big is a millimeter? C'mon, Rachel, speak English."

"Oh, a sixth of an inch, maybe. But it probably won't grow that fast."

"Better not. We're going to a wedding in New York the week before Dr. Mohs gets back. I'll plan to stop by on my way home."

"Do that. And have fun at the wedding. Don't worry."

Even after talking with Rachel, even on that glorious August day, I was still depressed. For the first time since that stretch when I was wearing the prosthesis, I was really down. But it wasn't just the skin cancer on my nose and the thought of a setback in my reconstruction.

Helen and Neil's wedding would be a real celebration. They knew our whole family, and we'd all been invited. Everyone was looking forward to one whale of a good time. But I felt an unsettling fear when I thought of seeing again all those New York friends, people who'd known me when I'd looked so different, when I'd worn most of my salary on my back and was certain I looked chic, attractive, and on some days pretty. What could they possibly think now?

A surprising, bewildering emotion welled up, almost choking me. I found myself mourning the loss of my former nose, much as I'd mourn the loss of someone beloved.

How shocking! Could I be this childish? Self-centered? Concerned with such a superficial thing?

While the rest of the country sweltered, a soft ocean breeze cooled my bedroom. Anyone with good sense would be up, not down, on a day like today.

But there was no one I could share my awful feeling with. Certainly not DeWitt. Since he'd favored my keeping the prosthesis in the first place—and it surely looked better than my present distorted beak—I didn't dare say anything.

Ellen was needlepointing in our family room with a childhood friend, Terri, one of our many visitors from the Middle West. I could hear their laughter mingling itself with the wind chime in the garden. How could I interrupt Ellen's good time to tell her how I felt?

And I knew if I shared my dismay with a close friend, she or he would simply feel compelled to bolster me with false compliments.

I was all alone, isolated.

So I drove out into the country and parked my car where I wouldn't be disturbed. I thanked God for therapy; this time I knew the right way to grope through the darkness and find the light.

First I allowed myself to break down and cry my heart out again. Then, feeling relieved, I tried to analyze what was at the root of all this agony. Was it because DeWitt would be ashamed of me at the wedding? No, I knew him better than that. Certainly I'd looked worse. Would my children be embarrassed? Of course not. All felt comfortable inviting their friends to our home, and going out with me socially.

I knew I wasn't being honest. My feelings had nothing to do with my family. What I was really wishing for was that my former friends would still find me attractive.

I was in the same predicament as a Harvard Business School graduate forced to return to his twenty-fifth reunion wearing a worn suit and frayed shirt and driving an old jalopy. I thought about his situation and tried to separate fact from fiction.

Fact was if he'd enjoyed close, warm friendships with class-mates twenty-five years ago, they'd be happy just to see him at the reunion. Fiction was his former friends would shun him; true friends don't do that. Fact was the reaction he'd elicit would be more favorable than that aroused by another classmate who arrived in a chauffeur-driven Rolls Royce, flawlessly attired in Bond Street clothes. The hardest thing to tolerate is not a friend's misfortune, but his sudden, overwhelming success.

Fact was I'd met with a mishap and my friends would be truly sorry it had happened. Fiction was they'd be more than momen-tarily concerned with my changed face. They'd be happy to be with me just as I'd be happy to be with them, no matter what hand fortune had dealt them.

This separating of fact from fiction threw some light on my problem. I drove home calm and secure, and with a certain pride. I'd turned the light onto my problems all by myself.

The dragon of deformity might occasionally raise his ghostly head, but I had him pretty well knocked out.

As I drove, I realized I had another problem, but there wasn't a thing I could do about it. Photographers had become the bane of my existence. And weddings had nearly as many photographers as presidential press conferences. At a social gathering I could feel great and forget my face until someone would drag out his camera.

It was strange.

In a mirror, my eyes seemed expressive, my hair still blonde and shining, my coloring attractive. But in a snapshot all I could see was a cadaver-like face with a twisted, misshapen half-nose. I looked grotesque. Then someone would rub salt into my wound when they said, "This is a good picture of you, Carolyn." Maybe for a medical journal it was.

If a face could break a camera, I felt sure it was mine. And if only it *would.* How I longed to grab every Minolta, Kodak, Nikon, Eastman, Polaroid, and Olympus and smash them all to smithereens.

At the wedding we greeted many old friends from the New York area. At the reception we hugged, we kissed, we reminisced. How glorious it was to see all those dear familiar faces after so many years away from New York.

My friends were still the same; I was still the same. Any self-consciousness about my appearance disappeared.

The reception was a true bacchanalian celebration. I became uneasy when I saw my young Ellen whooping it up with the rest of them, as though she thought bourbon were lemonade. Then I saw her waltzing away on that ballroom floor, her head held high, and my heart swelled with pride. I had raised a princess.

It was only when they took all those pictures that I felt anything but happiness. When the photographer appeared, I didn't just dislike him, I detested him. But I bit the bullet, and tried to keep any sharp silverware well out of reach.

When he said, "Now everybody smile," I became an actress. I smiled as I had never smiled before.

The whole week, I didn't give a single thought to the basal cell cancer on my nose. But on the plane to return to California with a stop-off at Dr. Mohs' office, I made up for lost time and worried about how large it would be. Surely *not* like the one on my *cheek.* I couldn't even bring myself to eat the airline's snack lunch. To make things worse, I traveled alone, because there was no reason for another member of our family to make the expensive detour to Madison for what might amount to only a thirty-minute procedure.

But on the plane I made up for lost time by worrying about how large it would be. Surely *not* like the one on my *cheek*. That trip became one of my dark valleys.

But Dr. Mohs found the cancer to be a small one. The third tiny slice came back negative. I walked out of his office and off down the hospital hallway.

"Free at last, free at last, thank God in heaven, I'm free at last!"

Every patient smiled, rejoicing with me.

14.

A NEW POSSIBILITY – PREVENTION

The cancer on my nose was tiny. But a few weeks later Dr. Mohs removed two malignancies on my upper lip. That procedure terrified me, and I sat limp through the whole thing. I 'd heard of several of his patients who, after losing some of their noses, had lost their upper lips.

The idea of my face without an upper lip sent shudders through my whole body. I tried to push the image out of my mind, afraid that just imagining it could make it happen. I'd heard they usually reconstructed an upper lip with cheek skin, but mine had already been used. What would they do then? I'd enjoyed a nice life with an imperfect nose. But without an upper lip?

I stopped playing golf, not wanting to risk sun, even with sunscreen and a hat. DeWitt was an avid golfer, and I relished the companionship of a mixed foursome. But giving up the game wasn't too hard to bear. I'd just as soon meet friends for a lazy, shaded lunch as try to whack my way out of a sand trap.

I'd once thought skin cancer only a nuisance. Now, finding a way to halt the curse of skin cancer became my most urgent concern. After talking with a student of mind control, I even tried her "scientific" approach. I closed my eyes and concentrated on my good cells destroying my bad cells.

While I was concentrating one morning, the telephone rang.

"Hi, Carolyn. It's Jeannie Marston. How are you?"

"Fine. And you?"

"Good. Are you and DeWitt free Saturday evening? Edgar and I want you to come to dinner."

"We'd love to. What time?"

"About seven."

"That'll be wonderful. See you then."

The usual small talk had already begun by the time we arrived. At the table, Jeannie seated me opposite Dr. Frank Dixon, head of Research Science at Scripps Clinic in La Jolla. In the candlelight, I felt I looked presentable. He probably didn't even notice my defective nose.

I hadn't met this doctor before, although his name was familiar. Unexpectedly, he leaned across the table,

"Why in the world don't you go to Dr. Edmund Klein in Buffalo and be cured?"

I nearly fell off my chair. "Cured?"

"Yes. I know Dr. Klein. He's helped many patients have fewer skin cancers, and in some cases no more skin cancers at all."

"But I'm a patient of Dr. Mohs in Wisconsin."

"Well, quit playing footsie with him and go see Klein."

"Is this the same Klein who was in a *Reader's Digest* article?"

"Probably. He's gotten a lot of media attention. A couple years ago he won the Lasker prize for combining immunotherapy and topical chemotherapy to treat skin cancer. He works out of Roswell Park, the large cancer institute in Buffalo."

"When I read the article I wondered how I could get to see

him. It sounded very promising to me."

"Ed Klein's a good friend. I'll give him a call and tell him you may be phoning for an appointment."

I smiled over at Jeannie, who was busy talking with DeWitt. She'd obviously arranged the dinner party so Dr. Dixon could tell me about Dr. Klein. He described Dr. Klein's treatment only briefly, but it was clear that it did indeed encourage good cells to devour bad cells.

The fear that had been haunting me since my last visit to Dr. Mohs dissipated as a warm feeling swept through me. I'd been shown the way to a doctor who was known for having rid people of skin cancer, using the body's own defenses. A loving God had moved me to Minneapolis so I'd get to Dr. Mohs in time. Now I couldn't help but wonder if this same Master Player had moved me to La Jolla so I'd be directed to Dr. Klein.

DeWitt and I both felt I should go to Buffalo.

But I thought I should touch base with Dr. Mohs. I called and told him that Dr. Dixon had suggested I see Dr. Klein.

"I think it's just as well to take your skin cancers off as they appear."

Damn. Now why would he say that? If a cure was possible, wouldn't he rather that I never got another cancer than to just nip it in the bud?

I took my problem to my local dermatologist.

"I'm familiar with Dr. Klein's work," Dr. Peters said. "Immunotherapy and surgery are both used to treat cancer. Why don't you use both? Klein's an honest man. He won't say he can help you unless he believes he can."

I made jokes about "shuffling off to Buffalo," which DeWitt thought were corny and Ellen didn't get. I shuffled off.

My first evening in Buffalo was fun. I flew across the continent and by seven o'clock that evening I was sitting in the Buffalo Holiday Inn dining room. My waitress was Shirley Rock, an attractive blonde, maybe forty.

We hit it off, and she joined me for an after dinner drink and lots of good conversation.

"I've come to see a Dr. Edmund Klein at Roswell Park Hospital. Ever heard of him?"

"Oh, of course," she said, "he's famous."

"They tell me he can help me have fewer skin cancers. A large spreading cancer destroyed the lower part of my nose. Now I'm having it rebuilt in Madison, Wisconsin."

"You don't seem self-conscious about it, are you?"

"Not as much as you might think, but I'll be glad when they get it finished."

"I think I know how you feel. I'm very sensitive about my false teeth," she said. "I've had them since I was twenty-one. My first marriage lasted five years. My husband never knew."

"Good heavens. That couldn't have been easy. How long have you worked here?"

"Six years. I had to get away from my husband; we lived in Rochester. Even my priest agreed I had to leave. But I had a two-year-old son."

"How'd you manage?"

"Father North told me, 'You go to Buffalo, get a job, a place to live, and find someone to look after Peter. I'll have the women in the parish keep an eye on things and see that Peter's okay. When you have things set up in Buffalo, call me and I'll set up a time when it'll be safe to come pick him up.'

"In two weeks, I had this job and a little apartment where the landlady could look after Peter. It was just hell when I took off, leaving him in Rochester. But now he's in third grade and doing great. I'm so proud of him."

Shirley pulled his picture from her wallet. A handsome boy. "Do you ever hear from his father?"

"Nope, not a word. I guess he thinks it's best this way."

She took a deep breath. "Now I'm going out with a swell guy, every Saturday night. He's sort of closed in, but I've got the whole week to think of nice things to say to him, you know, bring him out of his shell? What really worries me is what he'd think if he found out I had false teeth."

"How old is Mr. Saturday Night?"

"Fifty-five."

I laughed aloud. "Well, if he doesn't already have some false teeth, he soon will. My husband is his most endearing when he removes his false front tooth and makes a funny face."

"Well, have fun tomorrow with Dr. Klein. I sure hope he can help you."

From its name, I imagined Roswell Park Memorial Hospital would be either right in the center or on the edge of a park, with winding waterways and large shaded grassy areas. Instead, it was in a high crime area, surrounded by dilapidated houses, many evidently uninhabited, with broken windows. Tall weeds engulfed the yards and crumbling walks.

I arrived by taxi that first morning, and walked up a wheelchair ramp to the entrance. Later, a hospital employee cautioned me always to take a cab to and from the hospital, and never to use a hospital stairway. Security guards escort people to and from their parked cars.

Virtually every patient at Roswell has cancer. They are usually referred to Roswell only after treatment by other doctors has been unsuccessful. Most of the questions on the application form at the admission desk pertained to cancer. It was depressing to realize that other patients in the lobby could be fighting for their lives.

The décor was much like that of any other public institution. There were no carpets, as the floors were mopped and waxed constantly. Walls were sea-foam green, and all furniture utilitarian.

But paintings and drawings by local artists decorated the walls. Thank heaven someone had had the imagination to show this art. They made it a far more cheerful place. I saw a number of pink-smocked volunteers doing a lot of work, and I remembered my days as a volunteer nurse's aide at Bellevue Hospital in New York. Back in the forties, Bellevue was dismal. Never enough towels or sheets, and only one nurse for sixty patients. Somehow Roswell seemed much worse, simply because it was a cancer hospital.

"Most of these patients must feel helpless," I said, after I got directions from the head of volunteers. "I really admire your pink-smocked ladies. How can they take it, day after day?"

"You have it all wrong. When patients come here, most get a new treatment and take on new hope. One-third are cured."

I followed the green lines on the floor to the dermatology department, or Derm Clinic, and came to a construction site. The head of the volunteers told me they were moving the Derm Clinic. Partitions were going up, plastic sheets hung from the ceiling, telephone wires were strung everywhere and snaked across the floor. The hammering was deafening.

I walked up to a man in a white coat sitting behind a desk.

"I've come to see Dr. Klein," I yelled.

"I'll let them know you're here," he yelled back.

I went through the usual urine sample and blood-drawing routines. It took all my intelligence and agility to follow the instructions on the "clear catch urine sample" kit, while entangled in pantyhose. After they photographed me in the nude—an uplifting experience when everything's sagging—someone made six different skin injections on my forearms and pasted four cream-lined tapes on my upper arms. Each tape was labeled in code with a green magic marker. I was told to return the next morning to have them read.

It was close to noon, and I'd seen nothing of Dr. Klein. I wondered if he were only a fictional character around whom these medical exercises were structured. I went back to the Derm Clinic desk where I'd first reported in and asked when I could expect to see him.

"Go out to lunch and come back around two."

While waiting for a cab at the entrance to Roswell, I introduced myself to a Mrs. Malin. It turned out that she was also a patient of Dr. Klein's and staying at the same Holiday Inn. She suggested we share a cab. After a chat in the cab, we decided to have lunch together.

Mrs. Malin was a Liz Taylor beauty from New York's Park Avenue. Her gold jewelry made her a walking Tiffany ad.

"Two years ago I was diagnosed with a very unusual cancer," she said over lunch. "All the experts said I should have almost a quarter of my body amputated: a breast, a shoulder, and an arm, among other things. But they gave me no assurance the surgery would actually halt the cancer's progress. My closest friend kept insisting I avoid the surgery."

I looked again at her beautiful clothes and exceptional gold jewelry. My father had once told me never to envy anyone. I knew now what he meant.

"One day my husband and I saw Dr. Klein speak on TV about his treatment. He's an immunologist, but because he's primarily a dermatologist, he doesn't accept internal cancer patients unless they also have skin lesions.

"Cobalt had left me with skin lesions, and my husband was

determined I see Dr. Klein. He telephoned my cobalt doctor, whose offices were right across the street from our apartment, about getting me an appointment with Klein. But my doctor said he didn't think there was a chance of my seeing Klein.

"My husband is a very tall, strong man, and he raced across Park Avenue to this man's office. My doctor is quite small, and my husband lifted him right up by his lapels. Eyeball to eyeball, he ordered him, 'You get her to Dr. Klein.' The next day I was in Klein's office."

"How long ago was this?" I asked.

"Two years next month. You're here because of skin cancer?"

"Yes, I've had quite a lot of lesions."

"I think Dr. Klein will be the answer to your prayers. Skin, you know, is his main field."

She was planning a move to Florida, but still had to fight for her life.

She'd return every few weeks for treatment. "I don't care about the inconvenience. I feel like a different person. And my body is whole."

After lunch I checked in again at the Derm Clinic. "I'm here to see Dr. Klein about my basal cell skin cancers," I said to the woman behind the desk. "I hope he can help me."

"Oh, he snaps his finger at basal cell cancers," she said.

I sat down and opened my book to read, thinking, "Does this *ever* sound promising."

Around two o'clock that afternoon, there was an undercurrent of excitement, as though a head of state were approaching. Aides whispered, "He's come into the hospital." Others were murmuring, "He's on his way."

And soon after, late that afternoon, I was having a private consultation with this renowned doctor.

I found him very human. He had hazel eyes and sandy hair, which made him look rather young for his fifty-five years. Usually, I try never to talk with doctors, except as necessary. Whether he has six or sixty waiting patients, the last thing a doctor needs is a new-found chatty friend for a patient. But I couldn't stop myself. For some reason the words seemed to gush out.

"Dr. Klein, *you* are not saying this, *I'm* saying it: I'm *not* going to have any more skin cancers because I don't *want* any more." Breathless, I hurried on, "You see, sometimes I think God moves people across His chessboard just so they'll be in the right place at the right time."

I could hardly believe I had so shamelessly unburdened myself in my first brief consultation. I mean, that God seemed to be saying I needed to just meet the man. I felt very safe with Dr. Klein.

Dr. Klein smiled. "I believe I can help you have fewer lesions."

"Oh, wonderful."

He reviewed my medical history, which I'd written up and sent from California. "I don't want to start immunotherapy treatment until your nose is completely reconstructed."

"But that could be a year and a half from now. Shaping is going to proceed at six month intervals. In the meantime, I'll be a nervous wreck waiting to see if more skin cancer develops." To emphasize my predicament, I described the removal of cheek skin by the California doctor that turned out to be deep as the bowl of a teaspoon. Dr. Klein was sympathetic.

"If that's the case, then we can't treat you topically, with creams, because your lesions are too deep. From now on, go only to Dr. Mohs for any skin cancer removal. He's the best in the world."

He led me into an examining room where we were joined by several people on his staff. He put on a pair of rectangular, high-power magnifying glasses that stuck out about six inches in front of his eyes. A strong, hot light illuminated my skin.

"Here are the areas of Mrs. Shuck's face where large cancers have been removed by Dr. Mohs," he said. " She's presently having her nose reconstructed by a doctor in Madison." They all crowded around to peer.

"I'm hesitant to start immunotherapy treatment until her nose is completely reconstructed. Not that it would affect the reconstruction, but I don't want to be blamed if something goes wrong." He stood up and took off his magnifying glasses. "After all, Mrs. Shuck is primarily Dr. Mohs' patient."

That was certainly good to know, and I was sure Dr. Mohs would have appreciated it, as well. But there was only one thing I wanted to know.

"Do you think you can help me have fewer skin cancers?"

"Yes. I've treated many people who afterward had no more skin cancers. You wouldn't be number two and you wouldn't be number fifty."

I remembered my local dermatologist's emphasis on Dr. Klein's honesty. I couldn't wait to get things started. Perhaps his reluctance to do anything right away was because he didn't have Dr. Mohs' approval.

"Why don't you call Dr. Mohs? He won't be too surprised I'm here."

Dr. Klein left the room and I made small talk with his staff. He returned about ten minutes later.

"Just as I suspected, Dr. Mohs asked me, 'What are you doing with my patient? What are your statistics?'" His mouth pulled down into a grim line. He shook his head, looked glum.

"Be sure to have your skin tests read tomorrow, Mrs. Shuck. I'll see you then."

That evening I felt cold, then hot, then started shivering, as though I had flu. I crawled into bed and piled on covers. I slept well, but noticed in the morning that my forearms had some red swollen places where the injections had been made and my upper arms itched under the cream-lined tapes.

All teaching and research hospitals are alike. Staffs change constantly. But this one seemed especially disorganized because the Derm Clinic was being moved. When I found it the second morning, the place seemed deserted. A young woman in a white coat appeared. "Oh, hello. Why are you here?"

"I'm supposed to have my skin tests read."

She looked at my arms and peered closely at any place that had turned red or swollen. I'd never seen her before and had no idea if she were a nurse, an aide, a doctor, or secretary. All hospital personnel wore white coats, regardless of station.

"Well, I can't read these green markings. Who made the injections?"

I'd seen so many people the day before, I only knew it wasn't the photographer or the man who'd been installing telephones. "There must be some notations you can read. Maybe you can figure out the others, using the process of elimination."

"The injection needles are always in the same sequence in a tray; it's really just a matter of simple intelligence. I do know what they all mean."

Then why had they bothered to label my arms with the green marker, and warned me not to wash off the labeling? She jotted down some notations on a piece of paper. My chart wasn't there and I wondered if my test reactions would ever find their way to it. I felt as if I'd stepped through the looking glass into Immunotherapy Wonderland. No one seemed to be keeping track of a thing.

Then again, while everything was run with mechanized dispatch at that world-renowned clinic, the medical results had been disastrous for me.

Late that second morning my waitress friend, Shirley Rock, joined me for lunch in the hospital cafeteria. She'd suggested it the evening before, because she felt it might enliven my day.

"My biggest priority is to see my son gets through college. I have to put him ahead of everything." She smiled. "Even ahead of Mr. Saturday night." I just hoped the man she loved would wait for her. How lucky he'd be if he did.

That afternoon, I browsed through the hospital's medical library. I read a number of articles on Dr. Klein's work with skin cancer patients. Then I looked up some books on plastic surgery. The "after" pictures looked so much like the "before" pictures, I clapped the last volume shut and jumped into a waiting cab, to go look at something beautiful for a change.

Buffalo's Albright-Knox Art Museum was an oasis, with an outstanding collection, but the first thing I saw was a Grecian bust which had knocked about a bit over the years and lost—as you might guess—its nose.

A short block away was the city's historical museum. Fascinating. The city had been burned to the ground by the British in 1813. Only two buildings were left standing. From the little I'd seen during my short stay, the city hadn't renewed itself in modern times. I had the unkind thought that they needed to evacuate the place and have another good fire. Then they'd have a clean start.

Back at the Holiday Inn, I had a leisurely dinner, then went to my room to do a crossword puzzle and watch a little TV. Shirley Rock was off duty.

At nine in the morning of my third day in Buffalo, I returned to Roswell's dermatology department to have my skin tests read for the second time. There was more reddening and swelling, and the itching was worse. I was told to wait to see Dr. Klein.

Sitting in his hallway, I met many patients who had managed to get to him only because they had skin lesions. They had severe, life-threatening cancers. He was their last resort.

A beautiful woman, about forty, removed a metal tracheotomy tube in her throat, coughed, then replaced it.

"How long have you had your problem?" I asked.

"For five years," she said. "I turned every stone to get to Dr. Klein. Now I'm hospitalized because he's giving me a new treatment that might make my throat swell shut instantly. Still, if it can work, it'll be worth the risk."

Dr. Klein hurried through his hallway on the way to his office, but stopped to question her. She wasn't just an ordinary patient to him, one of dozens in the usual doctor's nine-to-five day. He couldn't have seemed more concerned if she'd been the only patient he had.

A spirited man who'd been out of the hospital on a pass sauntered into the hallway with a large sackful of canned beer. He acted as if he'd just blown in for Christmas Eve, his shopping done and ready for the party.

"He's pretty exuberant for someone who's hospitalized," I said to another patient.

"You should've seen him a few months ago," he said. "He looks and acts like a different person."

On the wall opposite my chair was a brass plaque. My eyes kept wandering back to it. "If I had my choice between a moon walk and the life of a single child with leukemia, I would never glance upward."

There was also a bulletin board on the wall with a news clipping tacked to it. Patients clustered around the bulletin board, read the news clipping again and again, and discussed it at length. The general feeling was that they had made it to a clearing.

Sobering as the afternoon had been, I had the feeling these patients and Dr. Klein were soldiers on the front lines of a battlefield, fighting not only for themselves but also for the men, women, and children who would follow them.

Finally, after eight hours of waiting, I saw Dr. Klein at five. His face was damp, some strands of hair plastered against it. I'd overheard someone say he hadn't been feeling well.

He looked over my face. "We'll be starting the creams shortly."

He handed me a commercial pamphlet on 5FU cream. "Look this over." "When should I come back?"

"Go home. I'll let you know."

As he dashed to the door, he stopped a nurse. "Give Mrs. Shuck some TB vaccine in orange juice. Oh, and give her some cortisone cream to stop the skin test reactions."

"What are the side effects of this vaccine?" I called after him.

"It's half the dose given a newborn baby," he shouted back.

But he'd said I couldn't have the creams. What was going on? Did he have me confused with another patient? I walked over to the nurse who stood by a refrigerator mixing some white powder in orange juice. She handed it to me and I drank it.

"Maybe you can straighten me out," I said. "Two days ago, Dr. Klein told me that he couldn't treat me topically because my lesions were too deep. Just now he said we'd start using the creams shortly. Wouldn't that be treating me topically?"

"Well, don't worry about any creams until he actually gives them to you." Her smile was reassuring.

"But I have no idea when I'm supposed to come back to see him."

"Don't worry about that, either."

I was still confused, but could only assume this world-renowned doctor knew what he was talking about. Jouncing back to the hotel in a dilapidated taxi, I read the pamphlet he'd given me about the creams. It claimed that 5FU could eradicate early basal cell cancers. But what would have happened if, instead of going to Dr. Mohs, I'd rubbed 5FU into the skin on my forehead, chin, and nose? Wouldn't I have soon been rubbing 5FU into bloody caverns, and been in one hell of a mess?

It was obvious Dr. Mohs was openly skeptical about my going to Buffalo. Going to that darn clinic for nose repair without Dr. Mohs' referral had been disastrous. What unseen danger might be lurking in this strange new medical world?

Arriving at the hotel, I felt faint, drained, in a state of emotional shock. I'd crossed the country with such high hopes. But I'd just spent three days in the hallway of a cancer center that seemed highly disorganized. Dr. Klein's last idea of what should be done for me was completely different from his first.

What a relief to see Shirley Rock on duty. I didn't even go to my room to freshen up, but took a seat at a corner table in the dining room.

"Please bring me a double bourbon," I asked her.

"No, I'll bring you a single. If you want another drink, I'll bring you one later." That's the kind of friend she'd already become, not eager to please me, just wanting to help.

"How would you like to meet me for lunch and do some shopping when you come back to Buffalo?" she asked later.

"Shirley, I don't know whether or not I'll ever be back. I don't know what's going on, but maybe Dr. Klein has to persuade Dr. Mohs his treatment can't hurt me, and might help."

"Oh, God," Shirley shook her head. "Doctors."

15.

MY CLUB

Back in La Jolla, I waited for a phone call from Dr. Klein. When I'd go out, I'd leave careful instructions with my cleaning woman to write down the telephone number of any caller. I was reluctant to leave an empty house, scared I'd miss the call.

Three weeks had passed since I'd been to Buffalo, and I'd almost given up. But one morning the telephone rang.

"Mrs. Shuck?" It was Dr. Klein.

"Yes?"

"Dr. Mohs agrees you should try immunotherapy treatment. I'll start your treatment here. When you go back to California, you're to stop by Madison so he can see the results."

"Oh that's wonderful, Dr. Klein. Great. When should I come?"

"Be at the Derm Clinic at eleven in the morning on October twenty-first."

"How long do you think I'll be in Buffalo?"

"Probably one day," I thought I heard him say.

I could hardly believe it, but I was too excited to ask him to repeat himself.

"Can my nose repair be continued?"

"Yes. That'll be okay."

I hung up, and dropped down on my knees to thank God. I felt safe undergoing this new treatment now that I knew a lifeline would be leading back to Dr. Mohs. My navigator had not abandoned me.

With that burden lifted, I began to look forward to my new trip, to seeing Shirley Rock and catching up on her life. She'd already told me in a letter that, just as I'd predicted, Mr. Saturday Night was having after-fifty dental problems, with under-the-gum-scraping, flossing, a water pic, the whole deal. After this recent trouble, he'd looked more closely at her teeth.

"Shirley, he'd said, "your teeth are beautiful. Are those front teeth real?"

"No, my front teeth are false."

She was getting braver.

I was sure I must have misunderstood Dr. Klein's remark when he said I'd probably stay only one day. Then again, maybe I had heard him correctly. Still, just to be safe, I presumed this first treatment would involve, at most, four days. So I took enough money and a few extra clothes in an overnight bag. But, instead of four days, I spent ten days in Buffalo. Because of the unsafe streets, I shuttled by cab between the Holiday Inn and Dr. Klein's offices, with my mobility thus as limited as my cash and wardrobe. During this sojourn and future visits to Buffalo, the Holiday Inn became My Club.

I can close my eyes today and be back, picturing My Club just as it was. Off the lobby was my usual spot, the dining room, which overlooked an almost always drained and barren swimming pool. But My Club seemed as glamorous as the Ritz's most elegant salon because it was so welcoming to me.

The floor of the lobby itself was a dark slate; the entrance was usually mud-tracked from the slushy outside snow. I still know just how that overstuffed black plastic and rust-colored furniture was arranged.

There was also that overstuffed taxi driver sitting in the lobby with his cap on, waiting for a fare. I was often it.

"How's your daughter, the one who lives in California?" I'd ask.

"She's great, and my grandson's playing little league. He's really good."

"Think you'll see them soon?"

"The wife and I, we'll probably drive out next summer, come June or July."

After four days, I ran into the glamorous Mrs. Malin. She'd come back from Florida for her immunotherapy shots.

"If I were you, I wouldn't go to Roswell until noon, at the earliest. Dr. Klein usually isn't there until afternoon."

So I didn't reset my watch, but stayed on La Jolla time, three hours earlier.

My days in Buffalo took on a pattern. I'd have breakfast in the coffee shop around noon, take a cab to Roswell, and sit in the hallway of the Derm Clinic waiting to see him.

The first day, he repeated the skin tests. Then he gave me two small tubes of white cream. "This one is 5FU, described in the commercial pamphlet I gave you, but one-tenth the commercial dosage, or less. The other is DNBC."

"How do I use them?"

"First moisten your face with water. Then apply them sparingly, doesn't matter which is first, one minute apart."

"What are they?"

"Chemotherapy medications originally used to treat internal cancer. We've put them in a cream base, the consistency of vanishing cream. They won't affect your normal skin. They only destroy precancerous tissue. You can wear makeup if you want to."

While waiting in Dr. Klein's hallway for him to read my skin tests or inspect my face, I read, knit on a sweater for Ellen, worked crossword puzzles, and chatted with other patients. I never knew what time I'd see him. Maybe two o'clock, maybe as late as nine.

Returning from Roswell, I knew Shirley Rock would be there to greet me at My Club. I'd always ask for one of her tables. Her hair was blonde and piled high. She's slim and beautifully groomed, and she sparkled. I was sure it was her smile.

All the men having Dinner for One hinted they'd like to talk with her. I didn't blame them; that's what I was waiting for too.

By the time I was seated in the dining room, I'd have spent several hours alone in Dr. Klein's hallway. On medical trips, my love of reading became priceless; I often would lose myself in a good book and enjoy the day. But in stressful situations, when I couldn't keep my mind on even a good story, I could manage to concentrate on a crossword puzzle. Anyone who's going to spend even a small amount of time in a hospital should be given an introductory book of them.

Still I could read, knit, or work puzzles only so much. With sixteen hours a day to kill, sometimes week after week, as I did in Buffalo, I was glad I grew up in a little town in the Southwest where, with nothing else to rely on, I had to develop a few diversionary skills of my own so that my imagination expanded with exercise.

During my business years at corporate sales meetings, I improved each salesman's appearance. I normalized his weight, performed plastic surgery to pin his ears back and adjust his double chins, and clothed him at Brooks Brothers.

At a church circle meeting I redecorated the hostess's house;

sometimes having to work fast to have the room completely repainted, slip-covered, and accessorized before the meeting was over.

At eye-glazing lectures, I stayed awake by putting the speakers through my spa. They emerged unbelievably chic.

When having Dinner for One, my favorite pastime was a game my mother taught me to play. When father was out of town, my mother and I would park on Main Street and imagine the life led by passing pedestrians. There were a variety of types in Bartlesville's sidewalk parade.

An Osage Indian from Pawhuska, nearby capitol of the Osage Nation, would walk by with his beautiful princess-like wife. He'd have driven over in their custom-built lavender Cadillac. Their son was studying law at Ann Arbor.

A young man was the young geologist just out of MIT, now working for a major oil company. He'd felt he'd come to the jumping off place, but he'd soon fall in love and like it out there.

It was easy to see the driller had just made a hit. We knew, because he, not his wife, was sporting a big diamond ring.

There'd be the ranch hand who'd come in for supplies. The worker at the local smelters. Eastern types whose families had blocks of oil company stock, and they'd come to actually see their investment. We imagined their lives as colorful, too.

Mother would only let kindness cloud her analysis when I hopped out of the car to join that parade, trying to look haughty, like a magazine model. I didn't walk far. I couldn't wait to get back to have mother tell me again how she would imagine my life if she didn't know me at all.

She didn't say she'd think I was a pimple-faced, skinny little seventh-grader, with tinsel-teeth braces aglow. Instead, I was just returned from my freshman year at Wellesley, where I'd been swept off my feet by several Harvard men, infuriating the son of the local banker and many other local lads as well.

I learned people placement from an expert. Mother could spot paste diamonds two blocks away—and a lot of other phony stuff, too—and she shared her secrets with me.

An unusual couple sat down one night in My Club. Two Boston Brahmins if I'd ever seen two. I could imagine them in a public dining room only in the Copely Plaza or, more likely, hidden away in a highly exclusive club. One look at the white haired mid-sixtyish lady, and I decided I'd like to look just like her. Aristocratic. And her pearls; a long plunging strand of them, and from their luster they were unmistakably real. When real pearls were less expensive, I told DeWitt I didn't care for them. Now that they were clearly out of sight and reach, I coveted them.

Soon a commotion started at the Brahmin table. Shirley was explaining that she didn't make the rules but they could speak to the manager. The manager came. They didn't look like trouble-some types. Were they asking for some exotic drink prohibited in New York State?

Later, I cornered Shirley. "What was that all about?"

"They insisted on ordering under-twelve-years-old plates at a dollar ninety-five. Little Jack Horner Hamburger or Tiny Tim Chicken, I think."

Was that how Mrs. Brahmin got her pearls? Maybe I didn't want any after all.

Staying at My Club was pleasant, but a bit confining. The only pain I ever suffered from Dr. Klein's treatment was self-inflicted burning eyes from reading, knitting, and crosswords. I played the Dinner for One game so many times, I became too good at it and had everyone in the dining room pegged even before I finished my salad. My stay would have to end sometime, but with absolutely no clue when that might be, I found the waiting that much harder to endure.

I found an idle typewriter at Roswell and wrote a letter to DeWitt, Ellen, John, Ted, and several friends. I knew I could make copies at the drugstore next door.

Dear Ones Out There,

Help! I'm a prisoner in a polka dot factory!

Two weeks ago, Dr. Klein called to set a date to start immunotherapy treatment in the hope I'll have fewer skin cancers pared away each year by Dr. Mohs. I'd asked Dr. Klein how long I'd be staying and thought I heard him say, "probably one day."

Remembering those skin tests took three days, I wondered how this could be.

But since I was to stop in Madison on my way back to California, I packed only a few things in a small bag I could tote on and off planes. That way my bag didn't end up in Atlanta or beat me back to California.

To travel in comfort, I wore wool knit slacks, a silk blouse, and sweater, so loungy for travel. On arrival in Buffalo, I found that instead of one bag, I had three: there was also a bag at each knee. My slacks looked like they'd come from the West Coast alone and had knelt all that long way in prayer.

Today is appropriately Halloween. After ten days, my two blouses are getting quite ripe, especially as I couldn't take a bath for three days while skin tests reacted.

On this day of hobgoblins and witches, I'm right in style with no effort. The bags at my knees are part of my costume. I can wear covering makeup over my red polka dots, but why waste it? I might run out just after spring, when I'm sprung.

Morning and evening I rub two creams into my first-dampened face. This causes pre-cancerous tissue to surface, making for many red dots. Twice a day I go to the hospital where Dr. Klein studies my face with his magnifying glasses while a bright light illuminates my surfacing red dots.

But Dr. Klein is determined, apparently, that they all come forward to disappear into the Nowhere. Just as some melt away, he maddeningly ups a cream dosage, which causes more and more to appear.

American Airlines now thinks Carolyn Shuck is a mythical figure or some lady making crank calls. I've made three reservations to leave; then canceled each. Red polka dots are finally fading to pink, but I'm certain Dr. Klein will prescribe yet stronger creams in his efforts to resurrect more. I'll be here for his observation . . . forevermore?

Oh, Dear Ones Out There, do not forget this prisoner at holiday time. Any small note of cheer or tiny gift such as soap flakes, deodorant, cologne, shampoo, cleaning compound, or CASH will be sincerely appreciated.

I dream now of snow falling, then melting away in the spring. Hopefully as the world turns, and summer arrives, I too will be Out There, free of red polka dots and with some skin left on my saved face.

Meanwhile, during the snow-filled winter, I'll spend idle moments negotiating with Yellow Cab to take Master Card. Do you suppose if I asked Dr. Klein for a loan he would let me go home?

Ah, a fond farewell from (take your choice):
Carolyn
Mrs. DeWitt Shuck
Your mom

I made my copies; but as it turned out, later that day I was given the okay to go home. En route, I stopped to see Dr. Mohs. He examined my face, measured polka dots, and wrote down their locations. He wanted to know if I later developed cancers in places where this treatment had forced tissue to surface and slough off.

I was relieved to find him his usual twinkly self.

"I'm glad you're willing to be a guinea pig," he said.

At home, I continued to apply the creams. One time I tried to count polka dots but lost track at five hundred. As some crusted up and disappeared, others continued to surface. Each week I reported to Dr. Klein. Using makeup, I enjoyed a normal life while engaged in polka dot manufacture.

In January, I went back to Buffalo so Dr. Klein could inspect my face. The polka dots had become even more numerous; in fact, I was covered with them.

Dr. Klein couldn't have been more excited. He ran over and kissed me on my splotched forehead. "Good heavens, a plastic surgeon could retire on you."

Then he took me into his office and studied my face with his magnifying glasses and hot white light.

"For every red dot we can see, there are invisible pre-cancerous cells this treatment is nipping in the bud. You have a *tremendous* immune system."

Three months later, my face was clear. It had been nice to carry on the polka dot production in my own cottage workshop. But I did wonder if they missed me at My Club.

16.

THE
VIRTUOSO
DOCTOR

D r. Klein was engaged in research and traveled a great deal, so
I could wait one, two, or five weeks to see him. He might call
me in California at one in the morning, Buffalo time, to tell me to
come back as soon as possible. If I were in Buffalo, maybe he'd call
me at Holiday Inn and say, "Hurry over to the Derm Clinic. I want
to see your skin tests."

"In the pitch dark? It's ten o'clock."

"Take a cab, of course."

But when I saw Dr. Klein, I knew he'd been worth waiting for.

Until he also had a private practice, three years later, I only saw
him at Roswell in the Derm Clinic. It was made up of several well-
lighted, well-equipped sections. They became almost private
examining rooms when white duck curtains were drawn closed.
Almost private. A person waiting in one section couldn't see in or
out, but could hear quite a bit. Of course I listened.

Dr. Klein looked on each patient as having a new and mysterious problem. He was as relentless as Sherlock Holmes, hoping to
unearth any obscure or overlooked clue that might help his diag-

nosis or indicate a shift in treatment.

"When did you first notice this swelling on your neck?" he'd ask.

"I don't know. Just a little while ago."

"Did you have it last week?"

"Oh yes. Before that."

"Last month?"

"Yes. I think so."

"Did you have it last Thanksgiving? Try to remember."

"Okay. Now I remember. I did have it then. I was getting dressed to go to my daughter's for the holiday. As I fastened my new blouse at the neck, I noticed the swelling. Yes, that was the first time I'd seen it."

"Was it as large then as it is now?"

"No. It's gotten bigger."

"At Thanksgiving, was it half its present size?"

"No, not that large."

"Was it the size of a pea? A marble? The size of a ping pong ball?"

"Just about the size of a pea."

"Did it itch? Was it painful?"

"No. I just saw it there."

After he heard a patient's description of his or her symptoms, Dr. Klein didn't classify them with a label, give them a number, and then run them through his medically computerized brain to get the treatment. He was a sort of virtuoso doctor, fine-tuning the exact treatment for each case.

During my first ten-day stay in Buffalo, he'd say to a resident, "Today I'm going to up the 5FU dosage and decrease the DNBC." It was as though he knew just when to tone down the cellos and bring the violins to a crescendo for the best effect. His form of medicine was a creative art.

My confusion during my initial visit to Buffalo stemmed from the fact that Dr. Klein sometimes mulled over a patient's case, verbally, right in front of the patient. He wasn't changing his mind about my topical treatment, just recounting his options aloud. I learned it was best to think of something else until he arrived at his conclusion.

Like any virtuoso, he was temperamental. His moods had wide swings. He could be glum, melancholy, and despondent one day; complaining, argumentative, and testy, the next. But more often than not, I'd see Dr. Klein jubilant, exultant, and in fine fettle. Despite his moodiness, doctors who worked under him weren't afraid to disagree with him.

"He can't *always* be right, can he?" I asked one of Klein's cohorts.

Shaking his head, he said, "Sometimes I swear he's clairvoyant."

I usually saw Dr. Klein in the late afternoon, but sometimes later in the evening. Time meant nothing to him. Security guards at Roswell told me he rarely left the hospital until after midnight, so I brought my knitting, book, and crosswords, and prepared to encamp. I didn't bring a sleeping bag, but one might have been useful. Some peanut butter and a martini would also have been nice.

On one trip, Dr. Klein saw me about four o'clock. The most recent cream application had only produced eleven red polka dots, quite a contrast to the hundreds during the first application. He said I was coming along nicely.

"I'd like to show you something," he said before he left the examining room. "Could you please stick around?"

After a long wait, I looked at my watch. Six thirty.

"Does Dr. Klein know I'm still here, or has he forgotten?" I asked his night secretary.

"Don't worry. He knows you're here."

I knitted and knitted until I came to a change in the pattern.

The instructions were back at My Club. I did the crossword. Read a few chapters. My eyes burned so, I knitted away with no pattern. It could always be ripped out.

Finally, at nine, Dr. Klein called me into his office. It was a cell. At most, it was ten by fifteen feet, with no windows. The walls were covered floor to ceiling with shelves jammed with stacks of bound papers and thick medical tomes. All I needed was a slight whiff to know they were mildewed, moldy.

"Have the photographer come in," Dr. Klein told his secretary.

After a few minutes the photographer arrived. "Show Mrs. Shuck the slides."

The slides pictured a woman's badly ulcerated back.

"Oh that poor woman," I said.

Then I thought of how I looked. No makeup, covered with polka dots, my nose still scarred and twisted.

"Well, I suppose she'd feel sorry for me, too," I said with a little laugh. Dr. Klein frowned. "Mrs. Shuck, it is *not* funny."

I straightened up in my chair and composed my face. More slides of the woman's back flashed on the screen, but in each slide the woman's back looked better. Finally, her back was clear and smooth.

Dr. Klein turned to me. "I cured that woman of an incurable disease in two weeks."

My heart jumped. Now, more than ever, I wanted to stay on his patient list.

"That is just fascinating."

He all but glared at me. "It is *not* fascinating. It is *awe inspiring.*"

It was hard, but I controlled myself. "Dr. Klein, I only have five adjectives, and I used my best one on you."

Although I've been confused, frustrated, even amused at times, I have tremendous respect for Dr. Klein's capability and enormous admiration for his relentless dedication. We've become good friends. When a dear friend was diagnosed with an advanced internal cancer and desperately wanted to find the best treatment, I put in a call to Dr. Klein. Within days my friend underwent treatment in Philadelphia that offered his best chance for a cure.

I was glad to reciprocate the favor when Dr. Klein needed a medication not available in this country. After an exhausting search through every back- road Tijuana pharmacy, Ellen and I got it for him.

Like all good friends, we teased each other. Since I'd never seen him at my appointment time, I asked, "How in the world did you ever make it through medical school, where you had to be at a certain place at a certain time?"

"Well, I didn't have any trouble getting through medical school, but I had a hard time getting a residency." I discovered his determination to do only what he wanted to do, when he wanted to do it, was known even then. But his medical talent outweighed his erratic behavior.

Like many doctors in those days, he chain-smoked. I once felt threatened while he examined me, when a long ash hung from his cigarette.

"Watch it, Dr. Klein. I heard you caught Mrs. Pearson on fire in her terry cloth robe."

He turned his head to one side in thought, then paused. "Come to think of it, I *still* owe that woman a robe."

Coming back from a trip to the Orient where we'd spent some time in Singapore, I'd applied his creams. I went back to show him the resulting polka dots. Singapore is on the equator so I'd ventured out to see temples and ruins protected by two sunscreens, a hat, and a parasol. But my protective ploys had failed. Instead of eleven red polka dots, my face had about sixty.

When Dr. Klein looked at the evidence, I felt as guilt-ridden as a child caught dipping into a candy jar. But Dr. Klein wasn't too upset.

"We all sin," he chanted as he marched down his hallway, "and those who sin must pay for their sins."

On another visit to see Dr. Klein, he again gave me the white powder in orange juice. Unlike my first visit, when I'd been so troubled when I gulped it down, this time I felt at ease.

"Why are you giving me the tuberculin vaccine, anyway?"

"It'll activate certain of your white corpuscles to manufacture lymphokines."

"What in the world are lymphokines?"

"They're substances that trigger the body's defense system. It's believed there are sixty to eighty of them. One of them is interferon."

"Oh, I've heard of that."

"There's some question whether it will prove as effective against cancer as against viral disease, but there are probably a lot of other lymphokines that will be far more effective against cancer."

"Why do you use DNBC in addition to 5FU?"

"They're more effective when used together than when either is used alone," he said. "The DNBC causes your own lymphokines to attack wherever a cancer cell is present, sort of like sending them on a search and destroy mission."

"When I read in the commercial pamphlet that 5FU could eradicate basal cell cancers, I was worried. With some of the large spreading cancers I've had on my face, couldn't I have been rubbing the creams into bloody caverns?"

Dr. Klein smiled. "No, we wouldn't let you do that. Should the creams turn up large cancerous lesions, we'd see Mohs surgery was used to remove all underground spreading extensions. Remember, the 5FU we're using is only a fraction of the dosage used commercially. The commercial dosage would burn up your skin."

I'd heard Dr. Klein and his associates were involved in research that could eventually help patients with deep-seated cancers, so I asked him what it was.

"Unfortunately, in patients with firmly established cancer, the body's defense system has been damaged. We're working on ways to repair the damage, using lymphokines. When they're injected into certain kinds of internal cancer that can show up in the skin, fifty-percent regress or disappear."

He showed me a picture of a woman who had reticulum cell cancer.

I'd never heard of it. "What is reticulum cell cancer?"

"A cancer of the white blood corpuscles," he said. "She was injected with lymphokines, and two weeks later the cancer had disappeared. Today, seven years later, she's still free of it."

"Good God. Do you mean to say this patient had cancerous cells in her blood circulating throughout her body—through her heart?"

"Heart, brain, lungs, liver, kidneys—everywhere."

"Can all cases of reticulum cell cancer respond to this treatment?

He sighed and shook his head. "No, but the fact that some do is significant." Then his face lit up. "Now, we're separating and studying the lymphokines individually." Maybe soon we'll know why some react the way they do."

The only critic Klein ever listened to was himself. If he'd always conformed to every rule of organized medicine, worked primarily for the acclaim of the medical hierarchy, spent energy pleasing every patient all the time, it's doubtful he'd have persevered in his research.

Instead, most of Klein's career has been devoted to research in cancer centers that were dependent on government grants. While I saw him at Roswell, I never received a bill. My treatment was experimental, and obviously supported by the taxpayers.

Despite his long hours and lifesaving research, Klein's income from Roswell was only a third of what a successful small-town surgeon makes. It didn't bother him until his children were ready for college. Then he set up a private dermatology practice in Williamsville, a Buffalo suburb.

"It disturbs me to shift some of my emphasis to earning money," he told me, "rather than confining my efforts exclusively to research."

"Why? Most doctors do want to make money. And after all your work, you deserve to make a little money."

"I guess it bothers me because of my rabbinical background."

It wasn't hard to tell how important he felt his research was. I'm sure he felt he was letting down all humanity by deciding to take care of himself and his family.

I tried on several occasions to get him to tell me about his early life. Because of his reluctance to talk about it, it took years for me to unearth the story.

Born in Vienna, the son of a poor rabbi, Klein grew up when Hitler was rising in power. At fourteen, he feared Hitler would soon take over Austria. So he applied for admittance to a London school. A month later he received an acceptance letter.

He told me of his harrowing escape to London, in the midst of the German occupation. Since he spoke little English when he arrived, he took shelter in a large vacant building for a time. Finally, he learned the school to which he'd been accepted was just around the corner. He graduated from this school, then won a scholarship, and graduated from the University of London.

A fifth column was operating in England, so he was sent to a refugee camp in Canada with many who spoke German. He applied to the University of Toronto. Accepted, he was released from the refugee camp. He worked as a lab assistant; his medical school fees were underwritten for eight years.

"The rest of my life has been pretty much the same. Every time a barrier has been erected and I've felt hopeless, a door has opened." He didn't say so, but I believe he feels he's led a charmed life.

No one else in his family survived the Holocaust.

17.

SAYING THE RIGHT THING

I spent many hours in Dr. Klein's hallway with a mother and her son, Pete, about twelve years old. The boy had a rare disease that kept them at Roswell for months at a time. Part of his lip had been removed, leaving him badly disfigured.

But Pete was cheerful, spirited, nice to be with. Sometimes he and I would stroll down to the news and sundries shop. Occasionally, I'd buy him a puzzle book. I'd watch him work the puzzles with spectacular speed and accuracy. Other patients and the doctors were always glad to have him around.

But everyone avoided the mother. She had no physical impairment, but was far more pitiable than her son. Her limp hair hung down, stringy, greasy. Always unkempt, she didn't seem to like herself much. But everyone avoided her because she was always criticizing and complaining. No doubt being away from her husband and other son for such long stays in Buffalo at Roswell only aggravated her unhappiness.

When I came into the hallway, she always managed to sit beside me and pour out her woes. I tried to escape by burying myself in a book, a crossword, or conversation with another patient, any patient. But each time she found me. Inevitably, she'd pull out her wallet to show me pictures of her other son.

"Now, he's just a beautiful boy," she'd say.

Since Pete was within earshot, I'd wince. It seemed she so desperately wanted to be identified with a handsome son that she couldn't help repeating her wallet and picture performance.

Once, when Pete was gone for a few minutes, she pulled out her wallet to tell me again about her beautiful son.

"Maybe it's not such a good idea to stress appearance so much," I said. "You probably don't realize how often you use the word 'beautiful' when Pete's listening."

"Oh, but I think Pete's beautiful too."

"Usually the word 'beautiful' describes appearance, not some inner quality. Maybe you ought to talk about Pete a little more. He's unusually bright, so I'd mention his intelligence. And what about his cheery disposition? Notice how everyone seems to like him?"

Of course, you can't tell someone anything unless that person is ready and willing to hear it. She was so preoccupied with her own problems that I'm sure what I said didn't penetrate her misery.

Soon after, I was called in to see Dr. Klein. "Why didn't you move away from that woman?" one of his staff asked.

"I couldn't. She's suffering. I think she needs professional counseling, and Roswell provides it."

The staff member shrugged and they continued with the exam.

"If that woman doesn't get help," I said, after everyone had looked over my face, "eventually she'll damn her child with an impairment far worse than the one you're trying to cure. A crippled ego is a lot worse than any other handicap."

My visit with Pete's mother made me remember things that were said to me after my nose became defective.

Some people always made me feel up. If someone invariably made me feel down, I'd simply avoid that person like the plague. Let them spread their gloom elsewhere.

These are just a few of the things said to me:

A three hundred pound friend, who gave no attention to her appearance, hugged and kissed me. "It doesn't matter what you look like," she said, "you're still a beautiful person inside." So well intentioned, her remark can't be classified as awful, but it's not among the best.

"My, but you have courage. Now, if it were me, I'd have to stay home because I'm so sensitive." This one was so bad it was hilarious. Since it was spoken by a woman I thought colorless, I wanted to say, "If I were you, I'd stay home, too."

"Lady, you're ugly." Kill the kid. No jury would convict.

"I'd just put a paper bag over your head." I'm not making it up.

"My aunt's nose was completely cancerous and they had to remove the whole thing. I won't go to see her, because I wouldn't touch a thing in her house." This was from a saleswoman in a Minneapolis boutique, who actually told me this after I'd asked to see a handbag in her display case. I was glad I'd taken psychology 101 and knew intelligence isn't distributed equally: for each very bright person there is one very stupid person. Fortunately for her, after I'd fingered the handbag, I knew it was what I wanted and I bought it. My guess is she either sterilized my money or just threw it out.

"I told you not to have that surgery; God, just look at you." This was before any nose shaping had been done. Did the speaker want me to lock myself in my room and do some serious brooding?

"It doesn't matter how your nose turns out. You're a very pretty woman." Even though she wasn't wearing her glasses, this person was on the right track. She, at least, made me feel better, not worse.

"Oh, hello. And did you notice the price of eggs in Safeway today?" My nose was still in a white bandage; didn't she notice that anything was just a little different? Still, her query was quite polite, and my feelings remained intact.

"What happened to you? What does the other person look like?" Fine, as it indicated the damage was only temporary, also that I had spunk and wasn't afraid of a scrap.

"It won't matter if the results of the surgeries aren't good. You have a fantastic personality." I predict a stellar career for the resident in plastic surgery who came up with this.

"Mrs. Shuck lights up the whole waiting room when she walks in." Dr. Davenport's nurse said this when I was wearing the prosthesis and was very depressed. I'd have lived on bread and water for six months just to hear that remark. It gets the A plus, as it complimented a part of me not related to my disfigurement.

I'm *still* living on that one.

18.

MEDICAL GODS
AND STRANGER
THINGS

By April of 1976 Dr. Davenport had shaped the earpieces and only needed to do one more touch-up. More important, I'd had no new skin cancers for almost two years. My efforts to save face were coming along beautifully.

It was then I learned I had to have a hysterectomy.

A swarm of butterflies invaded my stomach and set up camp there for the twenty-one days that snailed by before surgery. Not the graceful, pale yellow kind that delicately flit about, but the monstrous heavy-duty Monarch variety.

One reason for the raging butterflies was that DeWitt had been called back to Minnesota on urgent business. Our largest financial holding was in jeopardy, and its loss could have made life far more difficult for our whole family. He could only come back just before the surgery and stay only for the five days of hospitalization. So I put in a frantic call to Dr. Klein.

"I have to have a hysterectomy; they don't think it's cancer, just some abnormal cells."

"Who's your doctor?" he asked.

"Bill Lucas, right here at UCSD. He's supposed to be good, but maybe I should come to Roswell for another opinion."

"I'll check with our people, see what they say, then get back to you."

I stayed close to the phone all day. But it was eight in the evening before Dr. Klein finally called. "Our doctors say that if you're with Bill Lucas, they don't even want to look at you. They told me he's the best man on the West Coast, no one better anywhere in the country. You stick with him, and do *exactly* what he tells you to do."

My surgery was uneventful. Dr. Lucas assured me there was no malignancy. But instead of being on my feet a few hours after the operation, as I had been after plastic surgery, I felt as if I'd wandered into a pro football game and been dragged off the field with multiple injuries.

"Do you think I'll ever fully recover?" I asked Dr. Lucas when I got back to my room from recovery.

He laughed. "Better than most. But I want you to stay in bed for one whole month."

"Oh, don't worry about me. I don't do any heavy work. I have help three days a week."

"Up it to every day." He looked me right in the eye. "I want you to leave your bed only to shower, use the bathroom, and eat."

"Good night. Why? I know people who've gone out to dinner eight days after they've had their hysterectomy."

"Yes, but if you do as I say for one month, you'll feel great the rest of the year."

Two weeks later, at home, I took a look at my nose. *NO!* The skin on the tip was pulling up onto the bridge, and other parts were showing signs of slippage. My nose had become a mosaic. And just a month ago it had looked almost finished. Dr. Davenport had emphasized I'd have to keep my fingers crossed. Something had come uncrossed.

I stood back from the mirror. Oddly, I was not too unstrung. Convinced it was *my* nose, that *I* was in charge of its future, I knew the game was not over. The biggest card in the deck hadn't been played yet, and it was right there in my hand. The enforced month's bed rest was showing me that six weeks could pass in a hurry. As I lay there, obeying Dr. Lucas' instructions to the letter, I knew playing the ace of trumps—the forehead flap—couldn't be worse than the hysterectomy. The people on TV had become friends who'd still be with me and solitaire would still be the same game.

I'd miss Ellen bouncing in with her latest story, and no one could replace Ted helping me with the crossword. But nurses all have private lives I could surely unearth. And the surgeries would be good old plastic surgery, only skin deep, not the exhausting pro football kind. Within a day or two I'd be on my feet and feeling fine. Pooh. There'd be nothing to it.

And the time was finally ripe. That fall, Ellen would be far away in college, Ted even farther away in a New Guinea jungle, John launching a new career in New York, and DeWitt would be in Minnesota where I planned to join him.

While my family was busy, each doing his or her own thing, I could be in Madison, a short hop away from DeWitt, doing my own thing. I'd be giving up a tiny part of my life to attain a realizable dream. I decided to fly over to talk with Dr. Davenport the next time I went to Minnesota to be with DeWitt.

In June Ellen went off on an art tour of Europe with friends. Fully recovered from the hysterectomy, I tooled off to St. Paul, where DeWitt occupied a rented apartment.

I had my secret plan. One day, when DeWitt wouldn't be back until late in the evening, I drove to the airport and flew to Madison to talk to Dr. Davenport.

He shook his head when he saw the shrinkage of grafts. "A satisfactory nose cannot be made from the earpieces. Scar tissue from all the multiple grafts has pulled my shaping askew." He frowned, shook his head again, "What looked so promising has turned into a misshapen patchwork."

"Can you still do the forehead flap? I'm ready."

"Yes. It's the way I originally thought we should go." I thought he looked relieved.

He snapped a polaroid picture of my malformed nose.

"Do you think I'll like my nose as well as I did last March? Before it pulled out of shape?"

"I think you'll like it better. I can put some bone in the tip, giving you more of a profile, and your nose will be smooth."

He went with me to the appointment desk and placed the polaroid picture face up, where I couldn't avoid looking at it.

"The first appointment I can give you to start the flap is October sixth."

"But that's three months from now."

"The surgeries are so precisely scheduled, it's really the best I can do. You'll leave the hospital on November sixteenth. Sorry. I just can't do it sooner."

We made the appointments for the forehead flap surgeries, originally proposed five years before. I was stepping back in time to April 19, 1971, to the appointment I'd made for that scary surgery, to the day when my anti-perspirant had failed. But now I was extra-dry, cool, and calm.

Before going to the airport, I took a cab to Dr. Mohs' office. He found no new skin cancers.

"I've never seen your skin looking so healthy."

It was the only two year period in twenty-five years when I'd been free of skin cancer. I was thrilled.

Again a taxi sped me to the airport.

While I waited for my plane, I phoned Dr. Klein to tell him the good news about my clear skin.

"But my nose looks awful now. It's all pulled out of shape. I'm planning to have a forehead flap next October. Ever seen anyone who's had one?"

"Sure."

"How'd they look?"

"A hell of a lot better than you do," he said.

Just what I wanted to hear.

"You'd better get back here. I want to be sure all skin that's transferred from your forehead to your nose is fully immunotreated. I want to be sure it stays cancer-free during the surgery and afterward."

This time my wait was relaxed: no reading paragraphs in a book over and over, no waiting until the stroke of five to run into the airport dining room to order my martini. Now I bought a box of cinnamon Chiclets and a McCall's magazine, and settled myself in the familiar airport lobby.

I waltzed into the St. Paul apartment and announced my plans. DeWitt didn't echo my mood. "Carolyn, you are so impulsive and compulsive."

"Oh, c'mon . . ."

"You've had eight surgeries this year alone."

"Some were pretty minor."

"You've had five nose surgeries at the clinic, six earpiece surgeries with Davenport, and now you're going to try *this?*" he said.

My spirits sagged. "Look, I know I was impulsive when I

jumped up on the operating table at the clinic, but I've been thinking about the forehead flap for years. I didn't go to see Dr. Davenport without giving it plenty of thought."

"I think it's crazy."

"Remember the surgeon in San Francisco who said that the forehead flap is the *only* way to go, and it's not a dangerous operation?"

"I don't remember. The Carsons are picking us up for dinner in twenty minutes. You'd better get ready."

But before the evening ended, I made it clear to DeWitt that I'd never be satisfied with my patchwork nose, that I had to go ahead with my plans for the forehead flap.

"I'm just afraid it will risk your health, even endanger your life. You've already been through too much." DeWitt looked downcast.

"Dr. Davenport wouldn't do it if it were dangerous."

"I couldn't live without you, Carolyn. And I don't want the results to be disappointing to you."

"If they are, I'll know I tried my level best."

He pulled me to him, gave me a big hug, and kissed me. "I sure hope your dream comes true."

When I went to Buffalo to see Dr. Klein, he called together a group of plastic surgeons who practice at Roswell. All agreed a large flap was the way to go, but there were differing opinions as to where to get the skin. "I'd use a strip of skin from the collarbone," one said.

"A strip from her back would be better," said another.

A surgeon who had told me he knew Dr. Davenport shook his head. "No, only skin from her forehead will mold into a satisfactory nose."

But all felt none of these areas would be advisable, because they'd all been irradiated. The consensus was that X-rays had even penetrated to the skin on my back.

X-rays had gone clear through my body to the skin on my back? Strange I've never had any skin cancers there. Good heavens, is lung cancer next?

One plastic surgeon pointed to a thin-skin area on my back. "This has already been the donor-site for a graft."

"I was *born* with that area."

"Come back tomorrow at three," Dr. Klein said. "We'll tell you then what we think you should do."

The next day, about fifteen people in white coats gathered with Dr. Klein in a large consulting room. I felt like an accused criminal waiting to learn her fate from a jury.

"After consultation," Dr. Klein said, "the plastic surgeons and I have decided you shouldn't do anything about your nose. You have only irradiated skin to work with. We're afraid Dr. Davenport might bury some, making it unavailable to immunotherapy—and liable to sprout more underground skin cancer."

I made a face and stuck out my tongue at him.

"Carolyn, how would you like to spend six weeks having the forehead flap perfected, only to have to have it removed? It would be different if you were seventeen and looking for a husband."

My God. Were doctors, husbands, all men chauvinists? What does my marital status have to do with it?

"Besides, you might need your forehead skin later for reconstruction near the eye. We've been successful so far, but I'm not signing any papers."

I sat back in my chair, unable to sit upright any longer. Was I always going to look like this?

Judas. Talk about cruel and unusual punishment. These people had sentenced me to deformity prison—with no appeal. Stunned and dazed, my whole body was leaden.

"However," Dr. Klein said, "the final opinion on the matter will have to come from Dr. Mohs."

Thank God, I still had an appeal.

I jumped out of the cab that returned me to the Holiday Inn, crammed some money in the driver's hand, ran to the pay phone in the lobby, and used my credit card to call DeWitt. I couldn't wait for the time it would take to go up in the elevator and walk down the hall to my room.

"Oh, I'm sick." I was about to start crying. "Dr. Klein doesn't think I should have the forehead flap."

"I'd call Dr. Mohs. Do you have our credit card number?"

"Yes, that's how I called you."

"Let me know what he thinks."

I called Dr. Mohs. "I think you're being unduly alarmed about the X- rays penetrating to your back," he said. "No, I don't anticipate you'll have lung cancer. I'd go ahead and have my nose repaired if I were you."

I used my credit card again to get Dr. Davenport. "Have you done many forehead flaps using irradiated skin?"

"Yes—many."

"Have you ever had to remove one?"

"No."

"Have you ever had to make a major revision in one?"

"No, Carolyn, I've never had to do any of that."

"What would you think of using a back flap or a collarbone flap? Maybe it could eliminate shaving my head? Avoid the wig bit?"

"I'd never dream of using such tissue in the middle of your face; it'd be a blob, not shapeable."

"In my case, do you think there's a danger of burying irradiated skin?"

"Well, there certainly aren't any guarantees, but the risks are minimal, especially with the treatment Dr. Klein is providing."

Naturally, obviously, no doubt about it, I just *had* to call Rachel. Five years ago Rachel had told me that if anyone in the world could fix up my nose, Dr. Davenport could. She knew about everything that had gone on since. Now here I was, calling her from a pay phone in Buffalo.

"What alternative do I have?"

"Well, I guess you could wear Micropore tape on your nose for the rest of your life or maybe have another prosthesis made." Rachel knew I'd never accept either of those alternatives.

But I certainly didn't want to go ahead with this surgery if it meant Dr. Klein would abandon me. It had become as important to me to stop the skin cancers as to correct my disfigurement. I called him.

"Do you think this surgery would pose a major risk?" I asked him from the pay phone. "Getting my nose rebuilt is very important to me, Dr. Klein."

"Go ahead with the forehead flap, and we'll see what happens."

"I'm not sure I like the sound of that."

"If I thought it were really a major risk, I'd tell you to go get yourself another doctor."

Thank heaven he'd still continue my treatment.

Shirley Rock was pretty busy that evening, but I managed to talk over my dilemma with her during a lull.

"It's as though I'm dealing with medical gods. The gods of Remove and Rebuild are in Madison. It's the god of Prevention I've consulted here."

"I can see why you'd be confused."

"Well," I said, "it's obvious Dr. Davenport has reconstructed more noses with irradiated skin than the plastic surgeons at

Roswell. He refused to use back skin or collarbone skin, both of which they suggested—said you couldn't shape it into a good nose."

"You really have to grope your way through a maze, don't you?"

"You do. Trouble is, things aren't just black or white. You have to try to separate greater truths from lesser truths."

"I guess all you can do is go with your gut, and hope for the best."

I decided to cast my lot with the gods of Remove and Rebuild, and go ahead with the forehead flap surgery. And hope for the best.

I'd seated myself in the same corner of the dining room where I'd sat when I'd been so bewildered and despondent after my first visit to see Dr. Klein. Just because I could fly about on medical trips didn't mean I could do without a friend when I got there.

Friends like Shirley Rock.

I thought a lot that evening, as I watched Shirley waiting on tables, about what it must be like for people who haven't got a friend to open up to. It must be harder for men. Brought up to be strong and silent, no wonder some looked for their Shirley Rocks too.

What if I'd made it a point never to talk with a stranger? I wouldn't probably have survived the many trips to see Dr. Mohs, never knowing what he'd find to pare away. I've never told our children not to talk with strangers. Some day it may save their sanity. I've made marvelous friends of strangers. I thank God for them.

One seat-mate on a plane, a cancer patient, left me with the written note, "I have seen yesterday; I love today; I am not afraid of tomorrow."

On one journey I chose a seat next to a person with beautiful, long blond hair. When I sat down and looked again, I discovered fluffy blond sideburns. His corduroys were filthy. I decided to read my book, but curiosity overcame me.

"Are you going to LaCrosse, or on to Madison?"

"To LaCrosse. That's where my parents live. I left home during high school, couldn't get along with my folks. Thought I'd give California a try, but now I know I've got to finish my education. I think I have things worked out with my parents. Hope we'll be able to live together peacefully, at least for my last high school year."

We discussed some books. "Have you read *Catcher in the Rye?*" he asked.

"Yes, my son read it. I picked it up. Thought it provided a lot of insight."

"*The Agony and the Ecstacy?*"

"Quite a book. Took me time to get into it, but I was glad I kept going. You know, if you made it to California, I've no doubt some day you'll get to Italy. You'll have to see the Sistine Chapel."

"I plan to backpack through Europe, but not till I finish college. May take me several years, 'cause I'll have to work. But I want to get to know other cultures; how they've expressed themselves in different mediums."

I thought the young man perceptive and sensitive. Something told me he'd turn out to be quite a remarkable man.

We neared the airport. His foot was tapping the floor. "I've got butterflies in my stomach."

As we landed, I saw them standing there, right out of American Gothic. I knew there'd be fried chicken ready, no doubt apple pie too. From the looks of them, his parents were having butterflies too.

He stood up to deplane. "Have a . . . have a, a nice . . . the rest of your life."

Dear God, this is an important prayer. Please let those parents fill that boy with their love and understanding, not only with their apple pie and fried chicken. And, dear God, if you let them say one word about his hair or those cords, I'll be really mad at you.

I can remember when I was a small child, walking behind a man on the sidewalk, imitating his walk as perfectly as possible, so that maybe my mind would think exactly what his was thinking. It didn't work so I learned to devise other methods of finding out. I learned to soften and peel back the outer shell of every person I thought worth knowing, so I could savor their core.

During the 1940's I was out where the strangers are. It's been very important to me. By the time I lived in New York with a rotation of Vassar, Smith, and Wellesley graduates, I'd already savored the cores of doctors, nurses, shovel operators, executives, and secretaries. And I'd carried my lunch in a lunch box to a job in a tarpaper shack. I'd not only been living my own life; I'd lived the lives of many friends as well.

Out among strangers, I learned that entertaining people are wherever you happen to find them. I learned to appreciate choice people working in my kitchen; seated by them on a plane, at an exclusive dinner party, or a posh charity ball; or served by them in a motel dining room.

I learned a lot about people. The main thing I learned? We are all a lot alike.

The young women with whom I worked in that tarpaper shack were basically no different from those with whom I lived in New York. In those days, young women weren't too worried about careers. They had one big interest in life. Men. And because of their overwhelming concern with men, women had a lot in common.

They'd also been socially conditioned to be acutely aware of their appearance. So they tended to gather up their insecurities, and hang them on a defective physical feature, real or imaginary.

I'd always hung my insecurities on my thin-skin patches; Lula hung hers on her knees, which she claimed were strange; and Shirley Rock hangs hers right there on those dentures. Like every other person in the world, Shirley, Lula, and I are in some way insecure, vulnerable.

Appearance is more important to most women than to most men. But men are also vulnerable in their own ways. Many feel compelled to achieve some sort of status. Pressures on men are lessening, but unless a man is very secure, his worth in his own eyes is a reflection of how others rank him. But his status can often be subject to forces out of his control. Get a group of men working together—at the top of a corporate structure or on a shipping dock—and you've got politics. And the winds of politics can shift with no warning, increase to cyclone proportions, and sweep hard-earned status away.

The same thing can happen to money in an economic downswing—and for some men, their only worth is their "moneysworth." Laid off, capable men sometimes feel only shame.

Probably no person is so secure that nothing can shake him or her. We are all a lot alike: we are all vulnerable.

My medical trips could have been lonely affairs. DeWitt never failed to cross the country with me on medical trips involving surgery with anesthesia, but if he'd gone with me on every trip, I'd have become been a millstone around his neck. And a neck wearing a millstone soon has a pain in it.

But my medical trips were not lonely. Since I'd had practice making friends where I found them, I looked forward to some trips as adventures, where I'd get to know fascinating people in unexpected places. People who could help you sort out such complex issues as forehead flaps.

People like Shirley Rock.

19.

THREE LONG MONTHS

In June, when I'd made the appointments for the surgery, I'd been certain it was the thing to do. But because neither Dr. Klein nor DeWitt approved of my having the forehead flap, I became increasingly uneasy every time I thought of it. After all, Dr. Davenport *had* said not to go into it lightly. Now I had three long months to think it over.

In August, I left St. Paul for La Jolla. Back from her art tour, Ellen needed to pack again. This time she was off to Amherst College in less than a month.

I couldn't help mentioning my plan to close friends. "I'd never be so brave," one said.

Brave? I was terrified. Somehow I was running out of guts when I needed them most.

The retired California plastic surgeon who'd told me "The forehead flap's the only way to go" had also said, "If you decide to have it, don't discuss it with friends or family, only with a plastic surgeon."

This was invaluable advice, but I knew Dr. Davenport was

extremely busy with a number of patients. Still, one day I couldn't take it any longer and picked up the phone.

"Would you advise your wife, Marge, to do this thing?"

"Yes," he said. "I'd want her to look her best."

Every time I asked him a question, I got a green light and felt better, at least for a while.

The idea of a shaved scalp strip unnerved me, so I plunked down a huge sum and spent a lot of time getting a wig made to look like my real hair. It was now my remaining best feature.

I realized, but couldn't help it, that I'd built each of the three go-to-sleep surgeries for the forehead flap into mountains. I'd have to haul myself to the top of each one in my own tiny hand-operated car. But I knew that at each mountain peak, the merciful anesthesiologist would put me to sleep, and I could coast downhill until the next surgery.

If I could just make it to the summit of the first peak, I'd walk out of the Madison airport, the forehead flap behind me, with only two tinkerings to go.

My friends had lived through so much of my trouble, it had drained them of hopefulness. Like DeWitt, they felt I was compulsive about nose repair, if not completely out of my mind. After eleven failed attempts at a nose, why was I asking for more?

Was this decision just wishful thinking? An unattainable dream? Could Dr. Klein, DeWitt, and my friends all be wrong? Could only I be right?

Our children gave me the support I needed. Maybe the young are optimistic because they think nothing can go wrong.

Early that summer, before Ted left for two years in New Guinea, I told him of my plan. "You do what you want to do," he said after a tearful goodbye in the airport parking lot, "and when I see you again, you'll be beautiful."

Did he know how I'd cling to those words?

One day I burst into tears in front of Ellen. "I wouldn't have butterflies," she said, "I'd have bats whirling instead. But I'd still do it for a good looking nose that was my *own.*"

How wonderful to have a friend who understood. She knew I was afraid, but that I wanted my nose repaired.

By August, my tiny, deformed nose looked better and better to me. "I really think my present nose doesn't look too bad," I said to Ellen.

"Mo—therrr . . . ."

Just before she left, I looked at some snapshots. My whole face seemed deformed. "Would it really make any difference to have a nicer nose?"

Ellen shook her head. "That's like saying, 'I look sort of grungy today, so I'll never go to the beauty shop again or buy any more new clothes.'"

Do therapists need those degrees or are some just born with the skill?

My mind wasn't always on my nose during the three-month waiting period. DeWitt, Ellen, and I attended a wedding in St. Louis with all the accompanying parties. From there, we traveled on to deposit Ellen at Amherst.

I knew I'd miss her, but we could see she'd be happy with her new preppie roommate.

From Amherst I went to New York where John would soon start work as a neophyte lawyer. DeWitt would join me later in the week. That town was my oyster. I'd spent seven years there before marrying. I'd become a native, able to get anywhere on a subway, standing, with none of that sissy hanging onto the straps stuff. It was my old home town.

But when I checked into the Waldorf, I felt like a serf at the

Queen's palace. Everyone looked so "city," so affluent. My comfortable espadrilles weren't even California, they were Iowa. The lobby was full of people who seemed to know exactly what they were doing, and what they were doing was business, big business. Safely in my room, I called John, who hurried over. Just seeing him restored my self-esteem immediately.

So tall, handsome, so nearly Wall Street that no one would have noticed his worn L. L. Bean boots. I'd have been reassured to claim him as a distant relative, but here he was, my own flesh-and-blood. Imagine having been intimidated by those lesser beings in the lobby.

I needed a leaning post, and John was a sturdy one. "Ellen's told me you're nervous about your surgery. That's only natural, Mom, but it's definitely the thing for you to do."

New York took on a more prosperous tone as soon as DeWitt arrived.

John joined us for plays and dinners and the City was enjoyable as always. But soon we returned to St. Paul.

Surgery was only three weeks away.

We were living in a rented apartment, with only a coffee pot and maid service. We went out for dinner every night. I had nothing to do, twenty-four hours a day, but *think*.

I read, but with no comprehension.

If I only had a shut-off valve in my brain.

I tried to throw my thoughts out beyond the surgery—to visualize myself at the Madison airport, boarding the plane to St. Paul. The forehead flap's behind me. Only two touchups to go. If I could keep my mind filled with this vision, I could make it. It distracted me for a little while, but I couldn't keep it up for twenty-four hours a day. I'd soon be back in the rented living room, an open book in my lap.

At last the long wait ended. DeWitt and I went to Madison for the first surgery. Since it would only take an hour, I wasn't too fearful.

"What did Dr. Davenport *do* during the hour I was asleep?" I asked a resident afterward.

"He made an incision down the sides and across the bottom of the forehead piece. Then he lifted it loose from your forehead, but left it attached to your scalp. He played with it, making it into noses. After an hour, seeing that it didn't change color, he stitched it back down."

"Did he make it into noses to see if the skin was flexible enough?"

"Not really. He might have got an idea about the size and shape he wanted, but his main purpose was to see whether or not your forehead skin could survive for an hour with blood coming only from the scalp."

"He didn't have to line it?"

"Except for a small area, your nose already has a lining from your previous surgeries. In your next surgery, Dr. Davenport will line only a corresponding small area of the forehead skin with a little leg skin."

I was released from the hospital in two days, the left side of my forehead covered with a large piece of gauze. The stitches would be removed by a St. Paul doctor.

In one week, I would go back for the biggest surgery.

If Uncertainty, Apprehension, and Dread had been my companions before, now they brought along an army of kindred spirits. If I'd had to wait longer than a week, I'm sure I would've found some way to talk my way out of this surgery.

Only three months ago, I'd been relaxed when I'd chewed those Chiclets and read my magazine in the Madison airport. Now I was tormented. I'd talked with too many friends and seen them shudder. With my forehead skin "loosened," I was having second thoughts raised to the hundredth power.

Thank heaven it wasn't too cold or snowy in St. Paul to stop me from walking for miles. I remember every step of that path along the Mississippi, kicking the fallen rusty leaves, the wind biting my face and blowing my hair. I know how long it takes to walk to the stone bridge and back—forty-seven and a half minutes—and just where the tree roots stuck out above the ground so I had to step around them. I know because I took this blessed walk three times a day.

A Minneapolis friend made the forty-minute drive to see me for lunch. After spending so many days alone, I relished the temporary distraction to gossip about mutual friends. But how could I tell even this dear friend that I'd had the first stage of this surgery, but now was scared to death to proceed?

Certainly I couldn't mention my feelings to DeWitt. He'd have been overjoyed to have me stop while there was still time.

I kept hearing Dr. Klein's warning over and over in my mind: that the surgery could be dangerous if any irradiated skin were buried. Only two days before the big surgery, I phoned Dr. Davenport again about this possibility.

"Carolyn, that's *not* going to happen. Now stop having second thoughts." I felt a little better for a few hours, but his reassurance didn't dampen my fears for long.

Nights were filled by wide-awake visions of my shaved scalp, the scalp strip with the attached forehead piece dangling between my nose and ear. Every night I performed the surgery myself. I became an expert and could have done it in my sleep. But I couldn't sleep.

Finally, on the afternoon of October 13, I checked into the

hospital alone. I unpacked, donned robe and slippers, and for the thirteenth time gave my history to the thirteenth resident in plastic surgery. I felt more and more superstitious and more and more like an invalid.

I'd checked into the hospital alone because Dr. Davenport had taken DeWitt out for lunch. At first I presumed it was only a sociable thing to do since DeWitt was from out of town. But then I began to wonder, could Dr. Davenport be warning him of impending catastrophe?

When DeWitt got back, I found out Dr. Davenport had wanted to warn that I'd be a shocking sight.

He didn't have to warn me. I'd seen pictures and knew I'd look terrible-not just beat up with black eyes but unnatural, from-another-planet, terrible. I taped towels over the mirrors above the dresser and in the bathroom.

I'd leave it up to hospital personnel to look at me. I wasn't going to look at myself.

For my five-week stay, I'd lugged along books, robes, night-gowns, and thermal underwear. I knew this hospital could be chilly. I'd also brought along Christmas notepaper and green pens.

And I had that Japanese umbrella to hide behind. I'd designed it five years ago on the return flight to Minneapolis, after that first shocking proposal of the forehead flap. I'd sewn the vertical chiffon drop to the umbrella, black inside, white outside. I'd tested it out on my family. It worked well. While I carried it no one could see my face, but I could see out. And I'd embroidered the white chiffon with "HAVING A BEAUTY OPERATION—LOOK SIMPLY DREADFUL" in bright red. It would make it possible to leave my room and get exercise in the halls.

Night fell. I went to bed and played surgeon again. DeWitt was sound asleep at the Ivy Inn. Soon I tired of playing surgeon.

For the first time, I planned an exit from the hospital, never to return. After all, DeWitt loved me as I was, and friends didn't shun me. But I wondered what DeWitt would think if I appeared at the Ivy Inn with that huge trunk of a suitcase. He'd forever label me impulsive if I left now. And I thought of wonderful, persistent Dr. Davenport, and also the anesthesiologist who was fast becoming a good friend. At eight the next morning they'd be all suited up for surgery, scrubbed and germ free, and I'd not show up.

And I thought of how many people with far worse cancers never get a second chance. My thoughts became positive. "Just by checking into the hospital I've hauled myself more than halfway up the mountain to the biggest surgery. I can't stop now. I'll pull a little farther. Soon, Carolyn, you'll be at the summit where they'll say, 'Sleepy time,' and then, 'Wake up, Mrs. Shuck, your operation's over.'" Just one more exhausting pull upward and I'd make it to the summit.

I thought of Ted in the New Guinea jungle; how I wanted to look right the next time I saw him.

Of John, saying, "It's the thing for you to do."

Of Ellen when she told me, "I'd do it for a good looking nose that was my own."

And I thought of DeWitt and how he'd said, when he knew there was no changing my mind, "Carolyn, there's not one person in a million who could do what you're doing."

After all, I really did want to look as nice as I could for the rest of my life with him. I decided not to pack my bag and leave. I decided to live to be ninety and get my nose-worth.

I went to sleep.

20.

A MARTIAN

Poor DeWitt had no blindfold. Even though forewarned, when he saw me after the surgery, he was dealt an awful blow. He left my room shaking his head in disbelief, looking very sad.

"How *could* she let them do that to her?" I heard him ask a nurse.

By contrast, drifting in and out of the anesthetic, I was blissful because I knew I'd made it. My leg stung a little from the place where a thin layer of skin had been taken to cover the forehead and scalp areas, but nothing else hurt. I was coasting down from the highest mountain peak, exactly as I'd imagined I would after the hysterectomy. They'd said "sleepy time," and that was it. Nothing to it.

In a little more than a day I was enjoying a regular diet. They removed the IV so I could walk around. And yes, there was my old friend, Walter Cronkite, with the evening news. I wondered if he'd missed me the evening before when I was sleeping off the anesthetic.

I'd told Ted of my secret plan to cover all the mirrors.

He'd laughed. "You'll never last. You're more curious than anyone I know, except for Dad."

Ted was right. I didn't even make it past the second day. I peeled back one teeny corner of the towel covering the bathroom mirror, and peeked.

It wasn't so much gruesome as it was weird. I most resembled a Martian, dropped suddenly to Earth, caught, and scalped at the Battle of Custer's Last Stand.

A four-inch wide strip of shaved skin had been lifted from my scalp, one end still attached just above my right ear. The other end had become a continuous part of the piece of forehead skin, lifted from my forehead and now sewn to either side of my nose and around its tip. The shaved strip of skin lifted from the scalp had been tied into a narrow sort of tube, and swung down from above my right ear to my nose. I almost looked like an elephant scratching its ear with its trunk. Do Martians do this?

My eyes were discolored, swollen slits, peeking from behind the hanging strip. A blood splattered white bandage encircled my forehead and scalp. Sticking straight up from the bandage were bloodied patches of remaining hair. I was unrecognizable.

I could see why there was a "DO NOT ENTER—AUTHORIZED PERSONNEL ONLY" sign on my door. The hospital didn't want anyone to enter that room without sufficient warning, most likely to collapse on the floor. I could make for a lot of business in the cardiac ward.

Poor DeWitt. I'd wondered why he stayed only five minutes. Now I thought he deserved the Bronze Star for lasting even *one* minute.

I've always been repelled by gory sights because I can imagine the suffering and feel the pain myself. My appearance didn't repel me because I knew the terrible creature in the mirror wasn't feeling any pain at all. After two days, a resident told me I could take a shower and wash my hair. Wash my hair? I couldn't believe he expected this. All the same, I stepped into the shower and turned on warm water in a gentle stream. I let it spray on me, breaking its fall with my hands. Then I poured shampoo into my hands and made suds. I let a few suds fall on my head. It didn't sting; it was refreshing. I repeated the process, and for a long time let water splash all over my body.

It was nice to be clean, but it didn't transform me into a beauty. So my exposed scalp wouldn't show, a nurse brought a stack of flowered paper hats. But when I put one on, I thought it made me look even more ridiculous. It seemed a silly attempt to pretty-up a Martian.

One weekend, brave DeWitt was coming from his work in St. Paul. Preparing for his visit, I applied lipstick in exaggerated bow lips, rolled a white paper tube into a long cigarette holder, put on a flowered paper hat, and turned the brim up, flapper-fashion. I sat in a chair wearing a long silk robe, pulled up to bare my knee. When he opened the door, I pretended to smoke the fake cigarette and swung my leg. "Who do I remind you of?"

He knew immediately. I'd perfectly imitated an aging female relative. She'd lived in Hollywood and still mimicked movie stars of the twenties.

Every day I made myself write three Christmas notes. I gardened, trimming plants and soaking them in the bathtub. I've never been so clean. The minute I shed something, it was washed and hung out to dry. Doing chores first made watching TV more a diversion. I planned days around good programs.

Unfortunately, I couldn't read or do crossword puzzles. Even with a prescription lorgnette, I could only read for ten minutes, as the scalp strip covered one eye.

Truthfully, I've been more bored at other times in other places. My confinement was nothing compared with the boredom patients endure while immobilized for six weeks or more in traction.

A little boredom was nothing compared with the agony of the man and his wife who both knew she wasn't going to make it. Each evening, I met this man by the ice machine, and we had a little visit. I was carrying my light umbrella. He was carrying the heavy burden of knowing his wife was dying.

I'd use my ice to fix a bourbon that I could enjoy while listening to Walter. It made me feel less like a Martian.

Around ten every evening, when the halls were usually empty, I took my daily walks under the umbrella. Although no one could see my scalp or upper face, two small boys were a challenge. They sat on the floor and tried to peek. It required quick wrist action to tilt the umbrella down in their direction, then right it as I passed.

Walks became an entertaining pastime. One man apparently didn't read the "Look Simply Dreadful" inscription.

"Do you think it's raining?" he asked.

"I've felt a few sprinkles."

On one nightly walk, the halls were empty, even of nurses.

"Nurse, nurse!" I heard from a darkened room.

"I'm not a nurse, but I'll get one," I answered.

"I've got to throw up, but I don't have a basin," she wailed.

The nursing station was empty, so I rushed to her bedside, dropped my umbrella, thrust a basin under her chin, and muttered something about being deformed. Back in the hall, umbrella in hand, I waved for a far-away nurse.

In my room, I couldn't help but laugh at the woman's predicament. She must have thought she'd had an hallucination. Who receives nursing from a Martian playing the lead in Madam Butterfly? When I asked about her later, nurses told me she'd been moved to a lower floor because she was afraid of heights. No mention of a Martian.

When DeWitt left after one weekend visit, I felt a painful, stabbing moment of loneliness. Of course he telephoned every day, and I talked often with Ellen and John, but phone talks are just not the same as when someone is there with you. When a call came through from Ted on leave in Australia, I cried with happiness. But I recovered in time to reassure him and to confess that of course I'd peeked.

Many friends wrote, but Ted's letters were the most engrossing. Impeccable sources had told me Michael Rockefeller disappeared in Ted's very own jungle, and was thought to have been devoured by cannibals. Apparently, cannibals ingested those they admired. As Ted was both admirable and friendly with the natives, I'd sent this information to warn him.

"I know a very nice elderly man who once practiced canni-balism, but no longer does," Ted said. "Missing persons have prob-ably only been eaten by crocodiles. Our jungle is infested by them."

What a way to reassure a parent.

After I'd been a Martian for two weeks, twenty student nurses were assigned to our floor. Each day a new one cared for me. One amiable young woman offered to escort me when Dr. Davenport cut halfway through the scalp strip. This was done so the blood supply to my nose skin would not be removed suddenly. The little operation was to take place under a local in the Emergency Room downstairs.

Next morning, the young woman took me to Emergency in a wheelchair. I was *wheeled*, after doing two-mile sprints in the hall-ways. Nothing hurt, except the novocaine injections.

"Can you take Mrs. Shuck back by yourself?" Dr. Davenport asked after he finished the procedure.

"Look, I feel great," I said. "I'll be glad to wheel *her* back."

But I sat in the wheelchair as she pushed me onto the empty

elevator. "He asked that," she said when the doors closed, "because I fainted during your surgery."

The student nurses had never seen a patient undergoing the forehead flap, so their instructor wanted the four stages explained to them. Since I'd been good at demonstrating IBM machines when they were simple or lecturing at women's health centers, and because I'm a born ham, I volunteered to do the instruction. Why waste Dr. Davenport's time?

I was in my element and felt I did well behind the imaginary podium. But I was startled to hear my final words: "Now, are there any questions?" *What if there were one? I've told them all I know and probably added more.* But as fortune would have it, there was only a simple one about my leg skin.

As planned, one week after they'd cut halfway through the scalp tube in the Emergency Room under a local, they took me up to regular surgery, and gave me a shot. Again, they said, "Sleepy time," and I disappeared. When I awoke, back in my room again, I looked in the mirror.

The scalp strip was back in its home on my head, with stitches anchoring it there. The forehead skin, now upholstering my nose, was stitched down only across the bridge of my nose. Of course. That's where it *had* been attached to the scalp strip. The other stitches on my nose had been removed. A 2 by 3 inch scar on the left side of my forehead, where my present nose skin had been, was still covered with leg skin, thinner than the rest of my forehead skin. I could see that this scar could eventually be covered by a hair style like that of the wig I'd had made.

My hospital days were numbered. Only three days after the last big surgery, a resident told me I could wear my wig. I plopped it on quickly and sped out to lunch with a good friend. She happened to be in Madison and joined me, on the spur of the moment. We celebrated with two sherries. I was an Earthling again, nonchalant about the visible stitches across my nose.

Soon the day came when I walked out of the Madison airport and onto a plane for St. Paul. I'd pushed myself through the four surgeries. Only two tinkery nothings to go.

Finally, after six years, I had an *adequate* skin graft alive and well, and planted firmly on my nose. True, it looked as though I'd stuck my nose into a ball of pink putty, but I knew Dr. Davenport could shape it more like my former nose during that next year. He'd first lift up the left side of the skin graft and de-fat the underside. After he stitched that side back down, it would flatten and blend into my face. Later, he'd do the same thing with the right side. These were the "trimmings" he'd spoken of six years ago, when I'd been too terrified to ask what they were.

When I got to St. Paul, Thanksgiving was only days away. Ellen joined us there. Strange how these holidays always swung into place at exactly the right time. On a Halloween I'd been covered with pink polka dots. Now here it was Thanksgiving, just when I had so much to be thankful for. For DeWitt, for John, for Ted—and, I guessed, and for Ellen, even though she couldn't resist teasing me.

My comforting therapist for three long months before the forehead flap, Ellen had reverted to her silly old self. Seeing me without my wig, she accused me of having undergone a lobotomy.

I was especially thankful for the encouragement, the persistence, and the skill of Dr. Davenport. After the fiasco at the world-famous clinic, he was the hero waiting right there in the wings.

21.

YESTERDAY

By September of 1977, almost a year later, Dr. Davenport had completed the two "trimmings." My surgery was complete.

If it had been a movie, I'd have been propped up in a hospital bed, wearing a satin negligee and a marabou robe, my nose swathed in bandages. Then, on a long-awaited afternoon, Dr. Davenport would enter the room and slowly unveil my lovely new nose.

But this wasn't a movie. Instead, I was disappointed to see that my nose looked more like a potato than my original best feature.

When everyone said, "Your whole face looks better than it did before the forehead flap surgery," I wondered if they were only trying to boost my morale. Even bluntly-honest Dr. Klein thought it looked terrific. "What a masterful job," he said when he first saw it. "You just wait."

Wait? wait for what? It's all over. Have I accomplished my vow to look better than ever before? That silly vow I'd taken at the Ivy Inn on the day they'd started removing a lot of my nose. Hardly.

For the first time I couldn't console myself with the thought that I had only a temporary disfigurement. Anyone could see something had happened to my face; yet no further correction could be made. My long struggle was over, for better or worse.

No longer fighting my battle, I had a sudden retreat of the spirit. Not nearly so depressed as while wearing the prosthesis, still I was low and didn't know quite why. I went to see Dr. Maria Bowen again.

"Why do I feel depressed? I know I look better than I have since wearing the prosthesis. Even though my nose is not at all like I'd expected, it is my own skin. I know how it looks isn't *that* important, so why do I feel so let down?"

"I believe you're suffering a post-partum depression, similar to what many women experience after childbirth. It's just because it's over."

"Well," I said, "this is ridiculous. For years I've run about enjoying life with a noticeably flawed nose. I'm not going to let a nose that's a little too fat stop me now."

She smiled. "I very much doubt you will."

"Dr, Mohs' nurse, Rachel, has told me it takes a while for these forehead flap noses to flatten out and mold into the face. But it's been a year since the big surgery. Do you think I'm just being too impatient?"

"I imagine you are. Why don't you call her to see if you can expect it to flatten more?"

"That's a great idea."

I called her as soon as I got home. "Oh, sure," Rachel said, "just give it time. It's only been a short time since the last trimming."

What else could I do but simply wait? I became active and involved again, and my depression soon lifted.

I found new pleasure in walking the beach, learning more about bridge, having lunch with good friends, reading interesting books, and having more fun with DeWitt. Without the necessity for medical treks, we traveled to more exotic places. I had a great deal of pleasure in devoting my time once again to Planned Parenthood, an all-consuming interest since I started a clinic back in Keokuk. My mother was right. "The world is so full of a number of things, I'm sure we should all be as happy as kings."

But, you just never know what's going to happen next.

One evening a local plastic surgeon telephoned. "Mrs. Shuck, I'd just like to ask you one thing. How did you face the world so successfully with a facial deformity?"

I was startled. For a moment I didn't know what to say. "Why, I couldn't help it. That's like asking a four-year-old how he managed to keep playing, simply because he was missing his shoes and socks.

"Well, I work with a lot of patients who are deeply troubled by their facial defects. Try to think of things that helped you. Maybe they can help some of my patients."

Maybe they could. I gave it some thought, and in the end decided to write this book.

Right off, I knew it was far easier for me to handle facial deformity because I'd first coped with a bodily deformity. On Acapulco beaches, thin skin areas bared to the world, I often felt uncomfortable as though in the spotlight. I learned to imagine turning a real spotlight around so it shone on the other person.

In that way I became more aware of the other person's unimportant physical defects and important personal qualities. It's a rare person who isn't longing to let you know that he or she is important in some way. I found that, if I showed sincere interest, became a detective and asked penetrating questions, even the timid blossomed in my spotlight. Asked the right questions, even bores didn't stay boring for long. Used consciously, this device can help one develop a sincere interest in other people. Soon the conscious device isn't necessary; it's been replaced by an enjoyable hobby.

It was also easier for me to live normally despite my appearance because I knew with absolute certainty that being likeable was far more important than what I looked like. It was a conviction of which I was hardly conscious, because it had been there so long—ever since I'd entered a small co-ed college and embarked on my own personal study of what made young women popular. In that mini-society, I could do an in-depth study in short order. Within weeks, I'd observed that gorgeous young women often had unrepeated dates. Others less good-looking—and some quite homely by conventional standards—were quite popular with both sexes. Possibly the less attractive women were free to develop interesting personalities because they didn't have to maintain an "I am beautiful" image. Free to pursue ideas, hobbies, books, and causes, they had absorbing interests to share.

I was also fortunate to have worked for psychoanalysts when I first graduated from college. When I suffered my own severe depression, I knew you didn't need to be sick to make use of psychological aid; that to reach out for help wasn't a sign of weakness, but of strength. Even a mildly troubled patient would do well to talk things over with a professional before getting sicker.

I'd also discovered the benefits of exercise. Before my Saving Face adventures, I'd done exercises only sporadically, never taken golf seriously. I was one person who thought golf only a game, a thought that bordered on the sacrilegious to some of our friends. But when I began swimming to keep fit for repeated surgery, I found exercise helpful psychologically. It was something *I* was doing for my *own* rehabilitation. Within three days after surgery, I walked four miles about Madison and was exhilarated—as though I'd climbed Everest. Suddenly I was strong, powerful, proud. Moving the body relieves tension and whisks away mild depression.

By far the most important thing I learned about living with

disfigurement was that how others reacted to me was a direct
reflection of how I reacted to myself. If I seemed unconcerned
about my disfigurement, others were unconcerned. Friends and
family of someone with a disfigurement will be sorry, even grieved
that the patient has met with calamity. When he's obviously miser-
able, they share his misery, and can be enslaved by it. But when he's
happy, others are released to be happy too. Unsure of how to deal
with a medical situation, people naturally will take cues on how to
act from the patient.

At the same time, casual acquaintances aren't interested in the
details of how the injured party looks. When the patient is well
groomed and attractively dressed, he is telling the world that he
feels good about himself so that others can breathe a sigh of relief
and go ahead with their own pursuits.

People could easily see that my delightful friend Louise
Warren was not downhearted because she had just one leg. They
saw her whipping along with a red crutch when she wore her red
dress, a yellow crutch when she wore her yellow dress.

But she might not have been capable of this spirit if she hadn't
consulted a psychiatrist at one time.

Living with disfigurement often reminded me of playing golf
with a high handicap, something I did for many years. No matter
how many strokes a poor golfer has on a hole, no one is bothered if
he doesn't complain, holding up play. Should the poor player gripe
about every stroke, others players feel compelled to console him
with false compliments. Talk about annoying! Carrying another
person's ego for eighteen holes can get mighty heavy. Any golfer's
interest is in his own next putt, not in why someone else missed the
last one. And any player in the game of life has his own problems to
work out, and must be allowed the freedom to concentrate on them.

During the year of my major surgeries for the forehead flap,

DeWitt was undergoing his own suspense-filled year. It was crucial for him to be in Minnesota to keep our largest investment safe. He loved me and wanted me to be happy about my appearance, but his paramount interest had to be in keeping our income secure. I wanted him to concentrate on our financial future, not my nose repair.

During that same eventful year of 1977, John was launching his career in New York. Ted was acquiring the skills of a geophysicist, while living in a primitive jungle. Ellen was starting life as a college freshman, three thousand miles from home. They always expressed love and support, but each was naturally more interested in his own personal life.

In another conversation with the local plastic surgeon, he told me that some families and friends reject a person who becomes disfigured. This revelation made me sad.

Had my family and friends wanted to reject me? I didn't think so. How fortunate I'd been! Four family members and hundreds of friends and acquaintances, all of them accepting and supportive. How could anyone have such luck? The odds against it were greater than winning the lottery. Twice.

Suddenly, I remembered a statement I'd heard only that week: "The universe always agrees." I thought a lot about what that meant. Was the fact that I'd been accepted only an uncanny coincidence?

Over the years of disfigurement, I'd said to myself, "The world is an exciting, fun-filled place." And the universe had answered, "Yes, that's true." I'd also known, "Nothing has happened to the real inside me." And the universe had answered, "Yes, that's true."

Maybe sometimes when family members or friends reject a disfigured patient, it's because the patient has thought, "What a rotten, unfair world. Just look what's happened to me. I've become disfigured. Now I'm going to be rejected." If his world hears this refrain over and over, voiced aloud or repeated silently by his actions, his world will finally be forced to agree. It will answer, "Yes, that's true." He will be avoided. Rejected.

Shortly before a lot of my nose was removed, a Minneapolis acquaintance lost part of her lower jaw to skin cancer. Reconstruction hadn't been successful. When she and her husband had dinner at our club, the two of them always alone, my heart was heavy for her. It was rumored she'd become an alcoholic—easily understandable.

But when a similar thing happened to me, somehow it wasn't the same thing. It didn't even enter my mind that I lacked a proper nose when I called on a prominent businessman to solicit funds for Planned Parenthood. He received me cordially, and I enjoyed our short visit. I was concentrating so hard on my sales pitch that I never even thought about my face. Only three days later I realized, with amusement, that he must have wondered, "What *could* have happened to that woman's nose?"

W. C. Fields and Jimmy Durante couldn't help seeing comedy in their own outlandish noses. For many years I also had an outlandish nose. I didn't look at it and go into gales of laughter, but sometimes it was so inescapably ridiculous, so utterly absurd, I couldn't help laughing a little.

"Carolyn, you'd laugh if you were on a sinking ship," a friend once told me. It's true my ship was leaking a lot, and I was doing a lot of laughing. Others would say, "It's good you can laugh." It wasn't that I *could* laugh, it was that I couldn't help laughing. And laughter always put things back in focus.

Can there be a laughter gene one is born with? A bounce-back in the chromosomes that responds quickly to knockdowns? I hope not. I hope it's an acquired habit of looking back over your shoulder at yourself, and *having* to laugh.

Aren't we all a bit ridiculous from time to time?

22.

TODAY

How different today is, as I complete this saga in 2000. Today is golden compared with the traumatic days of that seemingly endless week when Dr. Mohs removed a lot of my nose; days following the fiasco at the clinic when I would shut myself in the bathroom and wail in anguish; leaden days when I thought I'd rather die than keep the prosthesis; the shocking one when a lot of my cheek was removed; that terrifying day when I discovered a cancer on the nose they were trying to rebuild; the bewildering days when I first went to see Dr. Klein in Buffalo. What a contrast my nights are now from those sleepless nights while waiting for the forehead flap, especially the night before the surgery when I all but left the hospital.

It's true I always rebounded rather quickly from those terrible days, and would find life once again full of its normal pleasures. But there were times when I went down into hell before I came back.

Today is a day for celebrating. Since starting Dr. Klein's treatment twenty-five years ago, I've had only three tiny facial skin cancers. I no longer wonder what part of my face will go next.

Undergoing his treatment, each of my basal cell cancers was halted right in the middle of a deluge. Starting in 1975 I saw Dr. Klein in Buffalo every two years and applied his creams for one month each year. Thank heaven I was willing to be a guinea pig.

God and Dr. Davenport must have had the same idea as to what sort of nose would best fit my face. Today my nose has settled in and, at a few paces, looks much as it did before this story began. When one chooses a surgeon of any kind, one should look for experience and skill in a specific procedure. But in choosing a plastic surgeon, one should also try for artistry, the good eye. I found both in Dr. Davenport.

Imperfections left from the clinic surgeries have largely disappeared.

Even for me, it's hard to believe I've had four major skin cancer removals, innumerable smaller ones, and eighteen reconstructive surgeries.

Did I ever get my face lifted? No. Enough of anything is plenty.

Today I don't need to go to Madison to see Dr. Mohs, the doctor who I believe saved my life. He's trained many dermatologists in Mohs' Micrographic Surgery. And those doctors have, in turn, trained others.

When he made a visit to California several years ago, we entertained him at a small dinner in our home. He told us, "I'm trying to get my congressman to have Hugh Greenway released from the Navy, I'm retiring to work exclusively on melanoma, and want him to come to replace me in Madison. He's one of the best men I've ever trained."

But Dr. Greenway chose to practice in La Jolla at Scripps Clinic. He has several examining rooms, technicians, assistants, residents-in-training, and a pathology lab at his elbow. Although I still deal with WALK–DON'T WALK signs, they're just part of the fifteen minute drive to his office. But there's no reclining barber chair, nor do I get to know wonderful strangers in his office. I'm in and out too fast.

A few months ago Dr. Greenway removed a basal cell cancer near DeWitt's eye. Novocaine was injected before each cutting, the common procedure today. The three necessary cuttings were done before noon. The same afternoon a plastic surgeon there repaired the damage. Based on data from many thousands of patients, the cure rate for Mohs' method is 99.8%. Today no other method approaches this dependability. The American Cancer Society endorses it as the most reliable method of removal. Only in rare cases are wounds not closed immediately.

This year I met a resident in Dr. Greenway's office who had come from Australia for training. He and I were talking about the thinning of the ozone layer which protects the earth from the sun's rays. This layer is now all but gone over the north and south poles.

"I've read that even here in southern California fourteen percent of the ozone layer's gone," I said. "One sunburns here much more quickly now than twenty years ago."

"In Australia, we're a lot closer to the south pole. The ozone layer is so thin there that school children are allowed to play outdoors at recess *only* if they wear long-sleeved shirts and wide-brimmed hats. If they don't have such clothing at school, they have to stay inside."

"Think that's what it's coming to everywhere?"

"Yes, and there'll be a lot more skin cancer. It's really important that people protect themselves with sunscreens."

"I slather it on every morning, even before I brush my teeth."

"That's the thing to do. There is no safe tan," he said.

"But how can enough dermatologists be trained in Mohs' surgery to take care of all the skin cancer?"

"Probably can't," he said. "But when a skin cancer *recurs*, it's especially important the Mohs' method be used. Using any other technique, the cure rate is at most seventy percent. Without Mohs' surgery, roughly one-third of these recurring cancers will continue to grow. Then the patient may have to go through an experience like yours."

I shook my head.

Recently, DeWitt and I had lunch with a friend of Ellen's whom we were getting to know for the first time. Ellen had probably told her about my experience with skin cancer. "Your mother is beautiful," the friend later said to our daughter. Ellen immediately passed the compliment along to me. Life itself has proved physical beauty an unimportant attribute, but because the comment would've been inconceivable for so many years, it was hard for me to hold back tears of joy.

"Someone sitting next to you might think, 'There's something strange about that woman's nose,'" Dr. Davenport had said when he first proposed the forehead flap. It's true someone scrutinizing my face will detect irregularities, but this doesn't worry me any more than an uneven hem worried me as a child.

I've always been a perfectionist about general effects but not details. In our home I want colors to be gloriously complementary. Cushions and flowers must always be a buttercup yellow, never a golden yellow, to complement french-blue carpets. But what's a little dust on the moldings? In clothing, I want cut, line, and color to be exactly right. But who cares if a few needle marks show in a let-out seam? And that's exactly the way I feel about my face.

What is vital is not your actual appearance. It's the way you feel about yourself. Self-image is a very important thing.

Men with facial disfigurement have an advantage. There's something masculine about men who have been scarred—German men are proud of those duelling scars. The man in the Hathaway shirt ad has a patch over his eye for a reason: on him it's sexy. On Madonna? No.

Everyone with facial disfigurement will react in his or her own way, but for me the mountain was there, and I had to do my best to scale it. If it had been impossible to repair my nose, I'm sure I could have accepted the inevitable and been happy.

How much better it would have been for everyone if I'd acted on my own feelings instead of trying to please others. Many times a gut feeling is the distilled essence of information a person has gathered. I should have trusted mine. I should have left Dr. Lang and his clinic after the failure of his first surgery and, gone back then and there to Dr. Davenport for the forehead flap. When I tried to please Dr. Lang by sticking with him, my face was badly damaged. Probably his reputation at the clinic was damaged as well.

When I tried to please DeWitt by attempting to manage with a prosthesis, I did him no favor. In the long run, he was forced to undergo even more numerous plastic surgeries with me.

How much better if I'd proceeded with the forehead flap immediately after the other surgeries failed. I thought DeWitt and my "significant others" wouldn't find the earpiece surgeries so frightening, but I should have turned down anything iffy and insisted on the forehead flap, which Dr. Davenport had twice recommended.

It's the patient's own responsibility to become well informed by specialists who have handled his problem successfully. Then he should make his own decision, act on it, and be willing to take the consequences. Others can't do this for him; they can't feel his feelings or read his mind. When I finally assumed responsibility for reconstruction of my nose, everything turned out well. But I was willing to face the consequences of failure.

I learned early that everyone is vulnerable, but during years of deformity I discovered that people are drawn to a person whose vulnerability shows. When people couldn't help seeing that I'd been wounded, I became desirable to have around. Both strangers and friends seemed free to open up, sharing concerns about children's divorces, husbands' retirement adjustments, their own fears and anxieties. I believe people felt safe with me.

During those years, I never had closer friendships, never enjoyed greater social festivity. When a resident told a nurse, "Mrs. Shuck wants to have her nose repaired so she'll be more socially acceptable," I thought that maybe I'd better not bother. If I became more socially acceptable, would I have to stop the world and get off?

My experience taught me other things which I'd never have learned otherwise. Regarding the loss of my nose—within that one week when Dr. Mohs pared a lot of it away—in the eyes of the world I gained a shiny, untarnished, brand new character. I'd lost a nose, but people instantaneously replaced it with a bright halo. Acquaintances suddenly imagined me uncommonly courageous, with marvelous spirit, and credited me with humor in the face of adversity. Some even thought me remarkable simply because I didn't become a recluse.

But I hadn't changed. I'd remained exactly the same, with all my strengths and weaknesses. DeWitt and I went along just as we always had: hugging a lot, loving a lot, and fighting a little. He didn't notice any halo; nor did my children or close friends. They knew me too well.

I talked about this phenomenon with my dear friend Louise Warren who'd become an amputee when she was eight. We agreed.

When a person continues to live normally, despite losing an appendage, having a serious illness, or becoming deformed in any way, the community often credits that person with a sterling character. It is one of life's little compensations.

She and I spoke of something else that automatically accompanies deformity. Anyone who is visibly different will be recognized and remembered for years to come by store clerks, beauticians, bank tellers, deliverymen, and social acquaintances, even if met only briefly and long ago. Not only was my visible difference remembered, so was my name. That quirk could put me at a disadvantage. Casual acquaintances would address me by name. Meanwhile, I'd frantically rummage through my memory for a clue as to theirs. Where *had* we met?

A woman's face is not her fortune. Her fortune lies elsewhere. We are only spirits going through a human experience, and human relationships are what count in life. When I was thirteen I went with my parents to the World's Fair in Chicago. My mother had a blister on her heel and wore a felt bedroom slipper. I thought she should have worn a gold mule, and I walked behind her so that no one would know she was my mother.

My children have never walked behind me; DeWitt escorted me gallantly everywhere. I think he cared less about my disfigurement than if his car had been wearing a crumpled right fender.

I can't believe it's now 2000, and I'm eighty. Just as was true when this tale began, I find it hard to believe my real age. Many times I still imagine myself twenty-one. But blessings accrue with age.

Recently, my friend Bunty said, "Carolyn, your face looks marvelous. Have you had more surgery?"

I laughed. "Heavens no, but thank you." I didn't say, "Your cataracts may be getting ripe for surgery; your eyesight is dimming." Can my own clouding cataracts be the reason my scars are diminishing? Is that why I'm looking better in the mirror?

This morning I bought what to me was an outrageously extravagant work of art: a heavenly garment made of old Brussels lace. In it, sitting in the lamplight ready to go out, I feel lovely and loveable, and very romantic.

For years I couldn't bear to look at snapshots. But this evening I'm wishing I had a photographer here—an artist with lighting effects so he could make me look like a Botticelli. It's not that I *am* beautiful. It's because after many difficult years, on this particular evening I'm *feeling* beautiful again. And feeling beautiful is every bit as good as being beautiful—probably better.

I could cry with happiness, but dare not let a tear roll down my cheek. We're off to dinner now with beloved friends, all with their own inside and outside faces, all going through the good and the bad in this life we share.

Today is just as I'd known it would be in the long, long ago. Tonight it will be easy come, easy go, and we'll all be laughing a lot. Everything has turned out just dandy because there's been a God who has always loved me. And the world has remained a delightful place where nothing too bad could ever happen again.

Nothing really too bad ever did.

EPILOGUE

My saga took place mostly in the nineteen seventies. Now, early in the twenty-first century, three of the doctors who helped me so much are no longer practicing medicine: Dr. Gordon Davenport, Dr. Edmund Klein, and Dr. Maria Bowen. Dr. Frederick Mohs is still associated with the University of Wisconsin Hospitals in Madison, Wisconsin. He is now concentrating his efforts on malignant melanoma. Other doctors trained by him are now doing Mohs' surgery there. Although the method he developed is recognized today as the most reliable skin cancer treatment, he has an open mind to possible new treatments for skin cancer.

To my knowledge, no one provides the same preventive treatment Dr. Klein gave me.

Dr. Bowen is dead.

As for the reconstruction of nose defects resulting from Mohs' surgery, your Mohs surgeon can probably recommend a plastic surgeon near your home who can do an acceptable and sometimes excellent reconstruction. This outcome is especially true if less than a major portion of the nose has been removed and the nostrils and tip are still intact.

The 99.8% five-year cure rate of Mohs' Micrographic Surgery is well established, based on statistics accumulated since 1936 on over one million patients. For this reason, reconstruction is rarely postponed. This means repair can be done before granulation (healing) takes place, making it much easier to get good results. Also, it is rare today that the reconstruction involves irradiated skin since for many years X-ray for acne hasn't been an accepted treatment.

Since I cannot breathe freely through the right side of my nose, I mentioned this to a local doctor who was removing my ear wax. On a visit to Dr. Greenway, I told him, "This doctor told me it would be a simple matter to open up my nostril."

"If anyone is going to touch your nose, it should be Dr. Gary Burget," he said.

"Where is he?"

"In Chicago."

Later Liz Sorenson, then about twenty-one years old, became Dr. Greenway's patient. She also became my good friend. Liz had a highly malignant tumor which made it necessary for him to remove a large portion of the side of her nose, as well as the floor and some of her upper lip on that side. Since the tumor was a rare and unusually malignant type of cancer, reconstruction was delayed while she wore a prosthesis.

When it was safe to do reconstruction, Dr. Greenway recommended she see Dr. Burget. A year later and frightened, she went to Chicago for the first surgery. In all, she made about five trips, alone, to see him. The results of her reconstruction were so good it still amazes me. Her experience with wonderful strangers was similar to mine. One summer she chose Chicago as her vacation destination so she could visit the good friends she'd made.

Later I saw Dr. Burget about my stuffy right nostril. In his waiting room, I chatted with one of his patients. Her entire nose had been missing and he'd reconstructed it. I couldn't tell anything had ever happened to it.

I decided not to do anything about opening up my nostril. It doesn't bother me enough to go through the major reconstruction Dr. Burget said would be necessary.

But I've become well acquainted with him. Because of my experience, he knows I'm interested in learning more about facial reconstruction. He wrote me, "Reconstruction of the face goes back 2,600 years to the fourth Veda of the Hindu religion. The forehead flap method arose somewhere in India around 1400 A. D., came to Europe in 1794." What sort of anesthesia was used—or not used? I shudder when I think of it. His letter continues, "Most noses, lips, and ears reconstructed over the centuries have looked more like garden vegetables than like the normal or beautiful structures we wish to achieve."

Together with Dr. Frederick J. Menick, a plastic surgeon of Tucson, Arizona, Dr. Burget has co-authored a textbook, "Aesthetic Reconstruction of the Nose." He lectures all over the world. Today, if I needed a major reconstruction of my nose, since Dr. Davenport has retired, I would beg, borrow or steal to get to Chicago so that Dr. Burget could do the repair. If my own doctor were reluctant to make an appointment with him, I could make my own simply by telephoning his office. His telephone number is easily accessible through Chicago directory assistance.

Today there is little excuse to let skin cancer grow to the point that mine did. Dermatologists who practice Mohs' Micrographic Surgery (chemosurgery) are located in nearly all major urban centers, all major cancer centers, and several foreign countries. The

American Cancer Institute rates it the most reliable skin cancer removal method.

Should you already have a dermatologist, if you have a recurrence of skin cancer tell him you want him to refer you to a doctor trained and experienced in Mohs' surgery. It is important that the Mohs surgeon be experienced in the technique, preferably handling at least five hundred cases a year. Be aware of your doctor's working twice on the same area, as this could signal a recurrence.

If you are prone to skin cancer, the most important thing you can do is to see your dermatologist regularly.

INDEX